CASE STUDIES IN THE
NEUROPSYCHOLOGY OF MEMORY

T0384880

Case Studies in the Neuropsychology of Memory

Edited by

Alan J. Parkin

University of Sussex, Brighton, UK

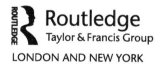

Taylor & Francis Group

LONDON AND NEW YORK

First published 1997 by Psychology Press Ltd

Published 2019 by Routledge
2 Park Square, Milton Park, Abingdon, Oxon OX14 4RN
52 Vanderbilt Avenue, New York, NY 10017

Routledge is an imprint of the Taylor & Francis Group, an informa business

Copyright © 1997 Taylor & Francis.

British Library Cataloguing in Publication Data

A catalogue record for this book is available from the British Library

Cover design by Peter Richards
Typeset by GCS, Leighton Buzzard, Bedfordshire

ISBN 13: 978-0-86377-507-9 (pbk)
ISBN 13: 978-0-86377-506-2 (hbk)

Contents

List of Contributors

James T. Becker, Neuropsychology Research Program, Departments of Psychiatry and Neurology, University of Pittsburgh Medical Center, Pittsburgh, PA 15213, USA

Ann D.M. Davies, Department of Psychology, University of Liverpool, and District Psychology Service, Wirral Community Healthcare, UK

Kim S. Graham, University Neurology Unit, Addenbrooke's Hospital, Cambridge CB2 2QQ, UK; and MRC Applied Psychology Unit, 15 Chaucer Road, Cambridge CB2 2EF, UK

J. Richard Hanley, Department of Psychology, University of Liverpool, Eleanor Rathbone Building, PO Box 147, Liverpool L69 3BX, UK

John R. Hodges, University Neurology Unit, Addenbrooke's Hospital, Cambridge CB2 2QQ, UK and MRC Applied Psychology Unit, 15 Chaucer Road, Cambridge CB2 2EF, UK

JC, London, UK

Evie Hughes, London, UK

Nicola M. Hunkin, Department of Clinical Neurology, Royal Hallamshire Hospital, University of Sheffield, Glossop Road, Sheffield S10 2JF, UK

Narinder Kapur, Wessex Neurological Centre, Southampton General Hospital, Southampton, S016 6YD, UK and Department of Psychology, University of Southampton, UK

Michael D. Kopelman, UMDS, Academic Unit of Psychiatry, St Thomas' Hospital, Lambeth Palace Road, London SE1 7EH, UK

Keith Laws, Psychology Department, University of Hertfordshire, College Lane, Hatfield AL10 9AB, UK

Katharine M. Leafhead, UMDS, Unit of Psychology, Guy's Hospital, London Bridge, London SE1 9RT, UK

Andrew R. Mayes, Department of Clinical Neurology, Royal Hallamshire Hospital, University of Sheffield, Glossop Road, Sheffield S10 2JF, UK

Peter J. McKenna, Fulbourn Hospital, Cambridge CB1 5EF, UK

Daniela Montaldi, Department of Applied Social Studies, University of Paisley, Paisley PA1 2BE, UK

Alan J. Parkin, Laboratory of Experimental Psychology, University of Sussex, Brighton BN1 9QG, UK

Karalyn Patterson, MRC Applied Psychology Unit, 15 Chaucer Road, Cambridge CB2 2EF, UK

Ella J. Squires, Laboratory of Experimental Psychology, University of Sussex, Brighton BN1 9QG, UK

Barbara A. Wilson, MRC Applied Psychology Unit, 15 Chaucer Road, Cambridge CB2 2EF, UK

1 Introduction

Alan J. Parkin
University of Sussex, UK

INTRODUCTION

I am not sure when cognitive neuropsychology was first used as a theoretical term, but I would consider the foundation of Max Coltheart's journal of the same name in 1984 as the first prominent use of the term. Since then there has been a minor intellectual revolution within experimental psychology, characterised by the use of individual case studies of brain-damaged people in the development of theories. Single case work is not new in psychology, but for experimental psychology it meant an important departure from the traditional group-based approach. Within the neuropsychology of memory the group-based approach had resulted in research being centred on the Wernicke–Korsakoff Syndrome because only here were there sufficient subjects available to form viable experimental groups—this is most aptly illustrated in the books by Talland (1965) and Butters and Cermak (1980). There were of course case reports, but most of these were clinically oriented. Only the pioneering work by Brenda Milner and her colleagues on the temporal lobectomy case HM resulted in single case data being used to support theoretical positions such as the dichotomy between short-term and long-term storage (Parkin, 1996a).

Within the neuropsychology of memory there has been an explosion of single case reports. The most important corollary of this is that the range of phenomena being demonstrated has grown immensely. In 1980 we were concerned with a few phenomena, such as release from proactive interference, and temporal gradients in retrograde amnesia. However, without

1

the need to create statistically acceptable groups it has been become possible to describe and publish far more types of memory impairment. This book contains a small snapshot of the kinds of study that have been fostered by the case study approach. As this introduction suggests, I would need a much larger book to cover the case approach to memory comprehensively. Instead I have asked colleagues to write chapters that each illustrate some facet of research that has arisen from the case study approach and, in this way, the reader can become aware that there is much more to the neuropsychology of memory than the amnesic syndrome.

The first chapter by Andrew Mayes and Daniela Montaldi perhaps takes us closest to the traditional concerns of amnesia research. These authors are involved with the relationship between structure and function. In the past this type of research depended on autopsy data but, as this chapter shows, it is now possible, via the use of neuroradiological techniques such as MRI and SPECT, to gain precise information about brain lesions and patterns of normal and abnormal activity in the living brain. This approach has confirmed much of what we have already assumed to be correct, such as the involvement of the midline thalamic structures in the generation of memory impairments. Beyond that, however, there have been some surprises, such as the differential involvement of right and left prefrontal cortex in encoding and retrieval respectively. Even more remarkable has been the discovery that a little-known parietal lobe structure called the precuneus appears to play a critical role in the retrieval of visual memories.

Kapur's chapter introduces us to a range of case studies all showing dramatic loss of autobiographical memory in comparison with often normal levels of performance on anterograde memory measures. Until work such as Kapur's highlighted these cases it had always been supposed that a dense retrograde amnesia would, inevitably, be associated with severe anterograde impairment and that relatively isolated retrograde amnesia should be attributed to psychogenic or malingered causes. However, as Kapur's series shows, this predominantly retrograde impairment can be associated with organic pathology, and it thus remains a challenge to accommodate this within a framework relating different brain structures to memory function.

Hunkin's chapter follows nicely from Kapur's by presenting perhaps one of the clearest examples of focal retrograde amnesia (FRA)—patient DH. However, although similar in many ways to Kapur's series, it is intriguing to note that Hunkin's patient does not have temporal lobe pathology. Rather he has lesions in the occipital lobes and the right parietal cortex. This pattern is also atypical of other reported cases of FRA in which there is usually involvement of the anterior temporal lobe but sparing of the hippocampal formation. This has led me to suggest that the typical FRA pattern arises from a functional hippocampal system attempting to recruit storage sites in a degraded   temporal   neocortex—the   outcome   being   below   average performance on anterograde memory tests (the content of which is soon forgotten) along with loss of pre-morbid knowledge (Parkin, 1996b). For Hunkin's case this explanation will not do and she offers an intriguing account based on Damasio and Damasio's (1989) multiregional retroactivation framework.

At first sight the chapter by Graham, Becker, Patterson, and Hodges might seem more at home in a set of aphasia case studies. However, cases such as the one they describe, GC, are of interest to memory theorists, for it has been noted that these patients have normal memory for the recent past despite impaired semantic memory and more remote memory loss. For me it is an intriguing question as to how they are able to have such good episodic memory when semantic memory is so badly disturbed—given traditional views that episodic memory provides a temporally based snapshot of semantic memory activity at any point in time. My second point concerns the relationship between patients such as GC and cases of FRA (see earlier). Both patient groups have temporal lobe damage with sparing of the hippocampus, which results in a reasonable degree of anterograde learning but marked remote memory impairment. Moreover, although not stressed, some cases of FRA clearly have semantic memory impairments. TJ (Kapur et al., 1994) for example, was unable to name any plays by Shakespeare despite previously being an English teacher. I wonder therefore whether the "semantic dementia" of the type shown by GC could grade imperceptibly into the FRA shown by TJ and, if so, what implications this has for the separability of episodic and semantic memory function.

Studies of the amnesic syndrome have consistently shown that both recall and recognition memory are badly impaired. The amnesic syndrome is typically associated with damage to midline diencephalic structures and the medial temporal lobe. However, early studies also suggested that ruptured aneurysms of the anterior communicating artery (ACoA) could also produce an amnesic state (Parkin & Leng, 1993). This was potentially interesting because disruption of this kind results in frontal lobe and basal forebrain damage. The chapter by Hanley and Davies emphasises that this early conclusion is incorrect and that the pattern of deficits exhibited by ACoA patients is different and of considerable theoretical interest. Their patient, ROB, performs normally on recognition tests, even though this demands contextual knowledge, but she performs very poorly on tests of recall. The authors argue for an "executive" contribution to memory which comprises both a retrieval component and a verification mechanism. They make a strong case that ROB has a retrieval deficit and point to other cases such as RW (Delbecq-Derouesné, Beauvois, & Shallice, 1990) as providing the other side of the dissociation—normal recall and impaired recognition.

My own account of JB, another man who suffered a ruptured ACoA aneurysm, provides a good contrast to that of ROB. First he is very much like

RW in that he makes very high levels of false alarms. His impairments are consistent with what one might term a verification deficit, but I develop this argument further and attempt to specify what this is in terms of underlying defective memory mechanisms. More specifically I show that JB's deficits stem largely from ineffective encoding.

Ten years ago the next two chapters would have been unthinkable in a neuropsychology textbook because their topics—schizophrenia and delusions—were considered part of psychiatry and thus not amenable to standard experimental investigation. In the case of schizophrenia that has all changed and McKenna and Law's chapter, through their account of SR, provides a very clear example of how memory impairment can lie at the heart of schizophrenia and that the disorder itself shows a range of memory deficits—thus offering up the schizophrenic population as a potentially rich source of dissociations. Moreover, this contribution introduces the reader to the deep divisions within psychiatry about the fundamental nature of schizophrenia—psychological deficit or brain disease? The chapter makes it clear that there is much to link the memory impairments of schizophrenia with those associated with particular brain pathologies and, as such, supports the notion of schizophrenia as a brain disease. Most notably SR has a "frontal" profile, in that she often performs disastrously on tests of frontal function as well as showing memory impairment on some tests. We have recently also noticed this in a case of atypical psychosis and speculated that the two factors are linked in generating memory impairment (Parkin & Stampfer, 1995) and that the deficit may have much in common with memory deficits associated with frontal lobe lesions.

The chapter by Leafhead and Kopelman concerns memory-associated Cotard's Delusion: the belief that one is dead. Delusional disorders such as this and others including Capgras Syndrome have, until much more recently, been viewed as unusual psychiatric syndromes. However, even here there has been change, with the realisation that cognitive analysis of these disorders can, at least in part, account for the deficits observed. In Capgras Syndrome, for example, it has been thought that right hemisphere lesions might contribute to the patient's misbelief that a close relative has been replaced by a double—rather like recognition without familiarity (Ellis & Young, 1990). But this view has now been moderated, in that Capgras is now seen as arising from an interaction of psychotic and cognitive deficits (Young, Ellis, Szulecka, & De Pauw, 1990). In line with this, Leafhead and Kopelman consider their patient's bizarre manifestations to be an amalgam of depressive symptoms, which, when combined with visual memory impairments, gave rise to disturbed feelings about reality.

The final two chapters consider memory rehabilitation, which, although gaining a much higher profile, still remains the Cinderella area of the subject. The two studies are greatly contrasting. The first, by Wilson, JC, and Hughes, is unique in two ways. First, it contains much material written by the patient himself and, second, it is the first detailed account of a patient evolving his own rehabilitation strategies. Presented in natural history form it shows how JC became more and more aware of his memory difficulties and accordingly devised strategies to deal with them. JC's story is, in many ways, every therapist's dream and, in reality, success of that kind will be a rare occurrence indeed. More typical perhaps is the case I studied with Ella Squires and Nikki Hunkin. Here we were confronted with an elderly somewhat obstinate man who, in stark contrast to JC, flatly refused to use any memory aids. Our account shows how even difficult patients like this can be educated by stealth to make use of memory notebooks. The study also provides an introduction to the method of errorless learning, which appears to show great promise in memory rehabilitation.

REFERENCES

Butters, N., & Cermak, L.S. (1980). *Alcoholic Korsakoff's syndrome. An information processing approach to amnesia.* New York: Academic Press.

Damasio, A.R., & Damasio, H. (1993). Cortical systems for retrieval of concrete knowledge: The convergence zone framework. In C. Koch & J.L. Davis (Eds.), *Large scale neural theories of the brain.* Cambridge, MA: MIT Press.

Delbecq-Derouesné J., Beauvois, M.F., & Shallice, T. (1990). Preserved recall versus impaired recognition. *Brain, 113,* 1045–1074.

Ellis, H.D., & Young, A.W. (1990). Accounting for delusional misidentifications. *British Journal of Psychiatry, 157,* 239–248.

Kapur, N., Ellison, D., Parkin, A.J., Hunkin, N.M. et al. (1994). Bilateral temporal lobe pathology with sparing of medial temporal lobe structures: Lesion profile and pattern of memory disorder. *Neuropsychologia, 32,* 23–38.

Parkin, A.J. (1996a). The amnesic patient HM. In C. Code (Ed.), *Classic case studies in neuropsychology.* Hove, UK: Erlbaum (UK) Taylor & Francis Ltd.

Parkin, A.J., (1996b). Focal retrograde amnesia: A multi-faceted disorder? *Acta Neuropathologica Belgica, 9,* 43–50.

Parkin, A.J., & Leng, N.R.C. (1993). *Neuropsychology of the amnesic syndrome.* Hove UK: Lawrence Erlbaum Associates Ltd.

Parkin, A.J. & Stampfer, H. (1995). Keeping out the past. In R. Campbell & M.A. Conway (Eds.), *Broken memories.* Oxford: Blackwell.

Talland, G.A. (1965). *Deranged memory.* New York: Academic Press.

Young, A.W., Ellis, H.D., Szulecka, T.K., & dePauw, K.W. (1990). Face processing impairments and delusional misidentification. *Behavioural Neurology, 3,* 153–168.

2 Neuroradiological Approaches to the Study of Organic Amnesia

Andrew R. Mayes
Royal Hallamshire Hospital, University of Sheffield, UK

Daniela Montaldi
University of Paisley, Scotland

INTRODUCTION

Research on amnesia basically involves identifying the patterns of memory and cognitive breakdown that result from brain lesions with particular locations. It has long been understood that this requires the development and use of hypothesis-driven memory and cognitive tests as well as the use of standardised tests and test batteries. But until the 1970s and the emergence of computerised tomography (CT), it was not feasible to identify the location of the lesions that caused the memory breakdown with any accuracy in life. Only if it was possible to perform a post-mortem analysis could the location of the underlying structural lesions be identified, and this could be decades after a patient's neuropsychological profile had been examined. Relatively few post-mortem anatomical analyses have been carried out, but those that were performed did indicate that particular aetiologies of organic amnesia, such as herpes simplex encephalitis and alcoholic Korsakoff syndrome, were associated with reasonably specific areas of brain damage, even though this brain damage was almost invariably not confined to single brain structures. Research on amnesia, therefore, tended to involve the comparison of patients or the study of patients in different aetiological groups, on the assumption that patients within an aetiological group would have reasonably homogeneous kinds of brain damage, and that the location of this brain damage would vary much more across, rather than within, different aetiological groups.

This "aetiological group" approach to research on amnesia has been used to specify the pattern of breakdown shown by patients with differently located lesions, and, where applicable, to argue that patients with differently located lesions have different patterns of memory and cognitive breakdown. For example, if post-encephalitic amnesics show a different pattern of performance from alcoholic Korsakoff patients, then it might be argued that medial temporal lobe lesions (found in post-encephalitics who have suffered from a Herpes simplex infection) cause a different pattern of memory breakdown from midline diencephalic lesions (the major lesion associated with Korsakoff syndrome). The strength of any such conclusion is weakened by two facts. First, brain damage even of patients with one aetiology is highly variable. For example, Herpes simplex encephalitis damage may sometimes be confined largely to the hippocampus, but in other patients a very large medial temporal lobe region may be effectively destroyed, and damage may extend to the orbitofrontal cortex and even into parts of the thalamus (see Mayes, 1988). Similarly, in Korsakoff's syndrome, damage to different thalamic nuclei is very variable, and to differing degrees can extend into other brain regions such as the frontal association cortex, basal forebrain structures, the hippocampus, and brain stem structures such as the cerebellum and locus coeruleus (and the hypothalamic structures to which it projects) (see Victor, Adams, & Collins, 1989; Mayes, Meudell, Mann, & Pickering, 1988). The second fact is related to the first, and is that most aetiologies are associated with variable degrees of damage to different brain systems. It is, therefore, difficult to be confident that differences in pattern of neuropsychological breakdown are related to particular kinds of selective brain damage.

With the emergence of better neuroradiological systems for measuring the structure and function of the brain, the problem of relating patterns of memory and cognitive impairment to the location of the dysfunctional brain regions responsible for the deficits has become much more tractable. It is now possible to image the structure of the brain in life using Magnetic Resonance Imaging (MRI) as well as CT scanning. With modern MRI systems spatial resolution is sufficiently good to enable structures such as the mammillary bodies and fornix to be readily imaged. Although not all forms of pathology produce images that contrast well with the images produced by corresponding healthy tissue, it is possible to use MRI scans to indicate exactly which brain structures are intact and which have received some degree of damage. It is also possible to measure the volumes of brain structures such as the hippocampus, and, by comparing these volumes with the mean and standard deviation of the volumes of equivalent structures in matched normal people, get a more precise estimate of the degree of damage. This has so far proved valuable in exploring the relationship between memory impairment and the location of brain damage produced by normal and abnormal ageing and by temporal lobe epilepsy (for example, see Lencz et al., 1992; Soininen et al., 1994) as the volumes of the left and right hippocampus and amygdala as well as of other structures can be correlated with the memory performance of patients.

In the last decade there have been considerable developments in the field of functional neuroimaging and its application to both the study of normal cognitive processes and the investigation of specific clinical disorders. The brain is an obligate glucose user and must metabolise this glucose aerobically, but has no stores of glycogen. Therefore, as all glucose and oxygen come directly from the blood, measures of regional cerebral blood flow (rCBF) reflect levels of brain activity. Positron Emission Tomography (PET), Single Photon Emission Computed Tomography (SPECT), and functional MRI (fMRI) all provide techniques for measuring brain activity. PET produces tomographic images reflecting the concentration of radioactive tracers in the brain. Using this technique, images can reflect the function of the brain in terms of glucose metabolism, oxygen uptake, or other functional parameters, depending on the particular technique used. SPECT imaging involves the intravenous administration of a radiopharmaceutical labelled with a gamma emitting isotope. The relative distribution of the isotope within the brain is then detected and reflects rCBF and, therefore, brain activity. Figure 2.1 (see Plate) illustrates the activity shown by a normal and a damaged brain as detected by SPECT. PET and SPECT approaches to neuroimaging are, therefore, in many ways similar. However, PET has one main advantage over SPECT, which is that it is capable of providing absolute values of brain activity while SPECT provides only relative measures of blood flow. The availability of PET scanners, however, is restricted on the basis of cost, as a cyclotron is required. Few medical centres, therefore, have a PET scanner, whereas SPECT scanning is slowly becoming a routine part of neurological and psychiatric investigations and, as a result, an increasing number of these scanners are becoming available. fMRI procedures have also been developed that enable levels of neuronal activity to be detected. The technique that has been most widely used to date is BOLD, which images blood oxygenation levels, but another technique, FAIR, is now also being used, which images blood flow into brain regions (Bandettini et al., 1995).

As it has been shown that the level of blood flow into a region and the level of oxygenation of that blood correlate well in both time and space with the level of neuronal activity, PET and SPECT can be used to determine whether regions that appear to be structurally intact are nevertheless functionally abnormal. Such abnormality might be found in brain regions that are distant from a structurally damaged region because they are no longer receiving appropriate neuronal inputs. This has been noted in patients who have suffered infarctions that have caused thalamic damage leading to amnesia. Although these patients usually do not have detectable structural damage to the frontal lobes, they often show reduced levels of metabolic activity in the frontal cortex and other neocortical regions when scanned in the resting state using PET or SPECT. For example, Levasseur et al. (1992) showed uniform cortical hypometabolism except in the sensorimotor cortex (which was unaffected) in a group of amnesic patients who had suffered bilateral paramedian artery thalamic infarcts. It remains to be established, of course, whether or not this widespread cortical hypometabolism played any role in the patients' memory problems.

Functional neuroimaging not only involves getting indirect measures of neuronal activity when subjects are in a resting state, it also involves getting such measures when subjects are engaged in specific forms of cognitive processing. This is sometimes referred to as the challenge technique. This technique involves either PET, SPECT, or fMRI being used to measure the location of the blood flow changes or blood oxygenation changes (and hence, indirectly, the neuronal activity changes) that are generated by specific psychological processes. In order to do this it is necessary to use a challenge paradigm in which the blood flow activity produced in a baseline state is subtracted from the blood flow activity produced in a challenge state. The intention is that the baseline and challenge activities should be identical except with respect to the psychological process of interest to the experimenters. This is a hard intention to fulfil and may require a series of comparisons of the challenge state with several baseline states. PET is the technique with the longest history in this area. In contrast, fMRI has the shortest history and hence there is still by no means universal agreement about how effective it is and what fMRI procedures are most appropriate in challenge studies. Subjects can be given repeated scans with fMRI because there is no evidence that MRI scanning is harmful, and up to 12 scans can be given with PET, whereas only two SPECT scans can be given in a short space of time—so SPECT can only be used to compare the activity associated with two different psychological states at most. But SPECT does offer a significant advantage over PET in the design and administration of cognitive activation procedures because the SPECT technique allows the task to be carried out away from the scanner in a less anxiety-provoking environment, while the PET technique does not.

Ungerleider (1995) has recently reviewed the literature relating to the use of PET challenge studies designed to explore the brain regions that mediate different aspects of memory (there have been very few such SPECT studies and fMRI studies are only just beginning). This research has been pursued in a number of different centres and there has been a reasonable amount of agreement between their findings. The part of the research that focused on the kinds of episodic and implicit memory examined in the study of amnesia has shown several things: (1) encoding activates particularly the left frontal cortex regardless of whether verbal or non-verbal information is being encoded, but not always the regions of the brain strongly implicated in amnesia. However, several recent studies have shown that encoding novel information or elaborative encoding of complex information can activate structures in the medial temporal lobes (for example, Grady et al., 1995); (2) episodic retrieval activates the right frontal cortex more than the left regardless of whether verbal or non-verbal information is being retrieved, and also regions in the posterior cortex such as the parietal lobes, the posterior cingulate, and the precuneus, but often fails to activate structures in the medial temporal lobes; (3) tasks that involve item-specific implicit memory (which was once called priming!) have so far, in every case except one (Schacter et al., 1995), found less activation in the brain regions where the primed information is likely to be represented, which is consistent with the notion that this kind of memory reflects more fluent processing of the remembered information.

Modern brain imaging techniques, therefore, allow the investigator to assess the location, degree, and kind of structural brain damage in patients who show relatively selective memory deficits. This is achieved through the use of CT and preferably MRI in most instances. Through use of PET, SPECT, and probably functional MR imaging in the resting state, it is possible to identify which apparently intact brain regions are nevertheless not working normally. Finally, by analysing memory challenge studies of patients in whom it is possible to match either encoding or retrieval performance to that of control subjects, it is possible to determine whether the underlying brain damage changes the way in which these operations are performed. Each of these approaches increases our ability to discover the relationship between memory deficits and specific kinds of brain dysfunction. The approaches will, however, be more likely to achieve this goal if patients with reasonably focal lesions are studied. In this chapter, we will illustrate this notion by describing a study we have undertaken of two patients with such focal lesions. One patient had a lesion of the fornix and the other had a bilateral thalamic lesion. We assessed these patients neuropsychologically, determined the location of their structural brain damage using MRI, and made a preliminary attempt to see whether they had similar functional brain deficits by performing an episodic retrieval challenge study using SPECT. As interpretation of the patients' performance depends on comparing them with normal subjects who show similar levels of retrieval, we will first outline the procedure and findings of the SPECT study as applied to a group of normal subjects.

A SPECT CHALLENGE STUDY OF EPISODIC
RETRIEVAL IN NORMAL PEOPLE

In this study, we used SPECT with technetium[99m]–hexamethylpropyleneamine oxime (Tc[99m]d, 1-HMPAO) to study the pattern of brain activation in two conditions in two groups of normal subjects. The conditions were very similar to two of the conditions used by Shallice et al. (1994) in a PET memory challenge study. In the baseline condition, subjects had to generate words that were semantically associated with high-frequency noun stimuli that were presented at a rate of about one every five seconds. In the memory challenge condition, subjects were required to recall the second word of a previously studied word pair in response to the presentation of the first word. The word pairs were weak semantic associates (for example, "stream–fish") and the stimulus words were presented at a rate matched to the baseline task. The intention was that the tasks would involve similar cognitive activities: crudely the baseline task would involve semantic retrieval whereas the challenge task would involve both semantic and episodic retrieval. Subtracting the activation produced by the baseline task from the activation produced by the challenge task should, therefore, reveal the brain activation engendered by episodic retrieval.

For the challenge task, subjects were trained on the target list of word pairs before the scanning was performed. The first group of six subjects comprised the high-performance group. This group was given sufficient training to ensure that their recall performance was 90–100% correct. The second group of four subjects was given less training and was tested at a longer delay so as to reduce their recall performance to between 50 and 60% correct. There were two reasons for including these two groups. The first reason was to ensure that the recall level of one group of normal subjects could be matched to that of a group of six amnesic subjects who were also included in this study. Matching retrieval levels is critical for such comparisons because if the levels were not matched, it could be argued that any brain activation differences between normal people and amnesics might have resulted from the fact that the amnesics were not performing the cognitive operations responsible for the brain activations in the normal people. If retrieval levels were matched, however, and brain activation patterns were different, then the amnesics would have to be mediating episodic retrieval in an abnormal way. The second reason for having two groups of normal subjects was to test whether the same mnemonic processes underlie the right frontal lobe activation and the more posterior neocortical activations produced by episodic retrieval.

Two co-registration procedures were performed, which we refer to collectively as the MRI–SPECT co-registration procedure. First, baseline SPECT images were co-registered with MR images. Second, challenge SPECT images were co-registered with baseline SPECT images, which also had the effect of co-registering them with the MR images. An automated procedure was used to achieve this, as it produced more accurate results than a manual procedure. There were two reasons why we used this MRI–SPECT co-registration procedure, which is illustrated in Fig. 2.1 (see coloured plate later in the chapter). The first reason was so as to identify better in which brain structures SPECT activation occurred. This greater anatomical precision was provided by the MR images. In contrast, SPECT images offer no precise structural information of their own. The second reason was that we wished to maximise the accuracy of the SPECT subtraction technique. The MRI–SPECT co-registration procedure aligns the baseline and challenge SPECT images more accurately than an equivalent SPECT–SPECT co-registration procedure. On a subject by subject basis, we then used the MRI scans to identify regions of interest (ROI) that previous PET challenge studies have shown are activated during episodic encoding and retrieval. To investigate possible differences between the two control groups, we followed a hypothesis-driven approach in which we compared the activation patterns (challenge state minus baseline state) in the frontal and posterior cortical regions that PET work has shown to be activated by episodic retrieval.

The comparisons revealed that the normal group with near ceiling levels of recall were more activated than were the group with relatively poor recall in the posterior cortex regions that included the parietal region bilaterally and the right precuneus. In contrast, the group with relatively poor recall showed more activation in the right lateral frontal region. This is shown in Fig. 2.2. We interpret this double dissociation in the following way: the activations in the posterior cortical regions reflect activity that occurs when memories are successfully retrieved. Future research will have to identify exactly what kinds of processing the activations are mediating, but there is good evidence that the precuneus activation mediates recall that involves the use of visual imagery (Fletcher et al., 1995; Shallice et al., 1994). When other factors are controlled, one would expect greater activation in these posterior regions when retrieval is more successful. The right frontal region activation occurs in a brain region widely believed to be involved with the planning of thinking processes. Parts of the frontal cortex are likely to play a role in planning the active search that is often necessary if retrieval is to succeed. This active search is likely to be engaged more fully by the group with relatively poor recall for whom the target items are presumably not readily available. The group with near ceiling levels of recall, however, is much more likely to find retrieval a relatively automatic process that requires little planning and active searching for target items.

The level of recall of the poorer of the two groups of normal subjects was quite closely matched to that of a group of six amnesics with a variety of brain lesions, whom we gave more opportunity to learn the target materials.

In order to determine whether the two groups might be using different brain structures to achieve similar levels of performance we did an exploratory comparison of the activation patterns shown by these two groups in anterior and posterior cortical regions. In the frontal region, the amnesics showed significantly more high left frontal cortex activation than the group of normal subjects with similar levels of recall, and less right frontal cortex activation (with even a trend towards deactivation). In the posterior cortex, they showed more right calcarine cortex activation. This latter difference we are unable to explain, unless it reflects an artefact caused by the exceptionally small standard deviation for the activation of the right calcarine region shown by the poorer performing normal subjects. Further work will be necessary to resolve this issue. There was also a trend for the amnesics to show more activation in the right precuneus. These differences are illustrated in Fig. 2.2.

The difference in the pattern of frontal activation shown by the amnesic group may be explicable. Although the patients' recall was quantitatively quite closely matched to that of the normal subjects, it may not have been qualitatively matched. Specifically, the amnesics may have been engaging in semantic retrieval (i.e. not recalling the item–context associations or not recollecting) and relying on episodic memory (i.e. recalling item–context associations or recollecting) hardly at all. This is consistent with Tulving's view (see Kapur et al., 1994; Tulving et al., 1994) that left frontal cortex activation reflects episodic encoding and semantic retrieval whereas right frontal cortex activation reflects episodic retrieval. Presumably, in normal people the right frontal cortex is activated by the limbic and diencephalic structures that are damaged in the amnesic patients. The trend towards greater right precuneus activation shown by the patients may indicate that they were more inclined than their control subjects to use visual imaging in their recall of the paired associate words (see Fletcher et al., 1995). This possibility can be directly tested.

Although all of the six individual patients showed the pattern of the whole amnesic group, there were also some differences, which are discussed in the next section where we describe two of the patients in more detail in order to illustrate the value of acquiring neuroradiological as well as neuropsychological data on patients.

CASE REPORTS ON TWO OF THE PATIENTS

Two of the amnesic patients had relatively focal lesions in different sites. Our MRI and SPECT scanning enabled us to obtain structural and functional images of their brains. We also obtained some further neuropsychological information from additional tests that we gave to them.

Patient RM

In 1989, RM, who was a 39-year-old postman, began to suffer from bad headaches. These became worse and more or less continuous over a period of several months and he began to develop memory problems. Prior to this time, his relatives report that he had had a very good memory. He eventually started to suffer from episodes in which he became unresponsive. CT scanning showed ventricular dilatation and a tumour in the anterior part of the third ventricle near to the fornix. This tumour, which was a colloid cyst, was surgically removed using a transcallosal approach that involves reaching the third ventricle by removing some of the overlying corpus callosum. Following his operation, he was described as remaining confused for several days, but was oriented by the time of his discharge.

At a neurosurgical outpatients clinic, three months after the operation, RM was described as having two problems. The first was that his previously excellent memory had deteriorated so that he was reduced to a state in which he had to write everything down. It was thought at that time that he would not be able to return to work at the Post Office because his job had required a considerable use of day-to-day memory. The second problem about which he complained was that he found great difficulty in crowds where there were large numbers of people talking because the distraction created prevented him from focusing his attention on the key elements of the conversation. In other words, he was complaining about finding it harder to concentrate when there was a high level of distraction. Despite the expectation, RM did return to work, although the rounds that he now does have been simplified to match his reduced levels of memory. The severity of the memory and attention prob-lems is reported to have remained unchanged since the operation.

FIG. 2.2.   (pp. 16–17) Three axial MRI scans (a) illustrate the ROIs investigated. The lowest slice (1) includes the following regions: Lateral frontal (FL); ventromedial frontal (VM); head of caudate (Dc); thalamus (Th); calcarine (calc); occipital (occ). The middle slice (2) includes: Lateral frontal (LF); cingulate (Cg); parietal (par); cuneus (cun). The high slice (3) includes; High lateral frontal (LFH); parietal (par); precuneus (PC).

Figures (b) to (d) illustrate regions showing blood flow changes where white and speckled areas indicate increased activation ($P < 0.01$ and $P < 0.07$ respectively) while striped areas indicates reduced activation ($P < 0.01$).

Figure (b) shows the results of the high performance control group and figure (c) shows the results of the matched (poor) performance control group. Activation in these two groups was compared using hypothesis-driven independent t-tests. Figure (d) illustrates the results of the amnesic group when compared to the matched control group.

It is important to note that the left-hand side of each scan corresponds to the right-hand side of the brain.

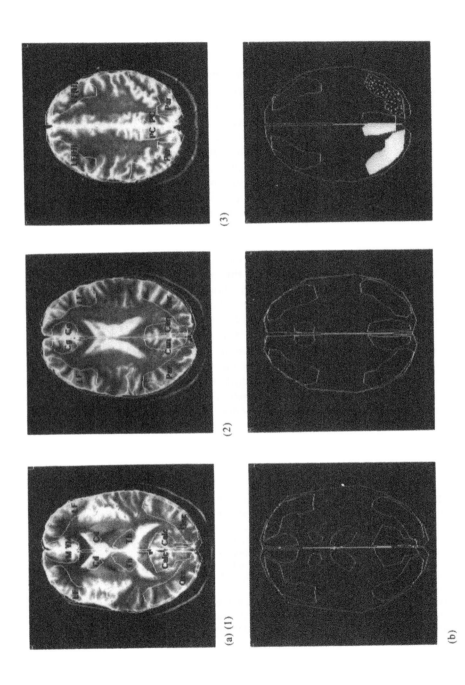

16

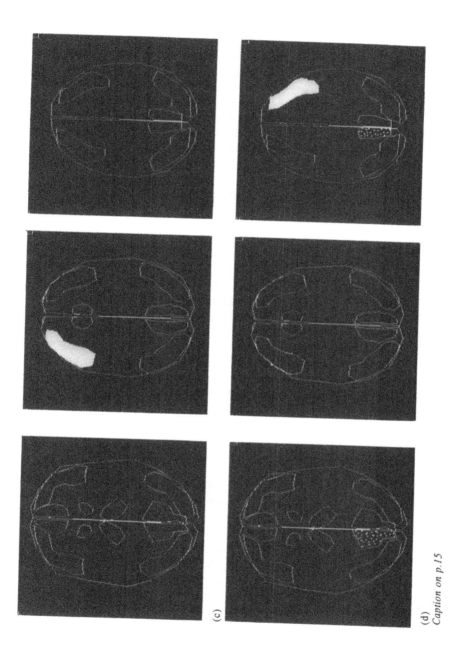

(c)

(d)
Caption on p.15

17

Careful inspection of our MRI scan of RM confirms that he has suffered relatively selective left fornix damage at a point that will disconnect the hippocampal direct projections to both the mammillary body on the left and the anterior thalamus on the left (see Fig. 2.3). There is, in fact, considerable atrophy of the left mammillary body, presumably as a result of the sectioning of the fornix. There is also some damage to the septum on the left and to the septal projections to the hippocampus that run in the fornix. The corpus callosum above the third ventricle has also been sectioned, but there has been no detectable damage to any other brain region, including all the regions such as the medial temporal lobes and midline thalamus that have been implicated in amnesia. The location of the damage on the left may to some extent be a reflection of the route of entry taken by the neurosurgeon.

It has long been argued that damage to structures in the classical circuit of Papez causes organic amnesia (for example, see Gaffan, 1992). In other words, lesions to the hippocampus, the fornix, the mammillary bodies, the anterior thalamus, and possibly to the structures to which the anterior thalamus projects, can each cause organic amnesia. More recently, a meta-analysis of many neuropsychological studies of amnesia by Aggleton and Shaw (1996) has suggested that hippocampal circuit lesions may cause an amnesia that does not have all the features of a full organic amnesia. They compared performance on Warrington's Recognition Memory Test (RMT) and found that there was a subgroup of amnesic patients who were not significantly impaired on this forced choice recognition test. These were patients who had relatively selective lesions of different structures in the Papez circuit. Although they performed better on this recognition task than the other amnesics, they performed no better on recall tests taken from the Wechsler Memory Scale–Revised (WMS–R). If correct, this suggests that damage to various parts of the hippocampal circuit, including the fornix, may cause less of a deficit in forced choice recognition (at least at short delays) than in free recall.

Two patients, who, like RM, had colloid cysts, underwent a similar operation to remove them, and suffered fornix damage as a result, have been described by Hodges and Carpenter (1991). Although both verbal and non-verbal memory may have initially been equally impaired, the patients showed selective improvement in their non-verbal memory in the period of two years (case 1) and one year (case 2) following their operations. CT and MRI found that the left fornix had been dissected as would be expected from the selective impairment in verbal memory. In case 1, however, both fornices appeared to have been severed, but, in case 2, damage was confined to the left fornix. As, apart from severance of the overlying corpus callosum, no further brain damage was detectable, the relative lack of impairment of non-verbal memory in case 1 remains a puzzle.

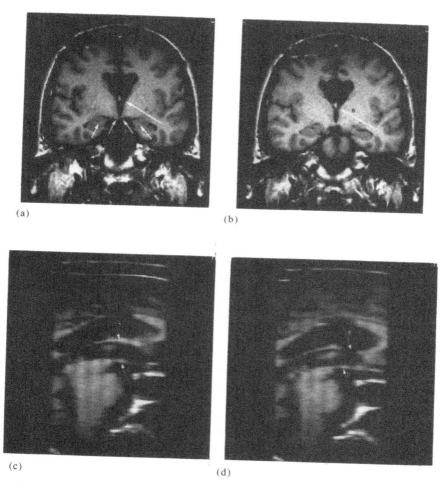

(a)

(b)

(c)

(d)

FIG. 2.3. Coronal and reconstructed sagittal scans illustrating left-sided fornix and mammillary body damage in RM.

Figures (a) and (b) show left fornix damage [A,B] as well as left mammillary body damage [D] relative to the right [C]. Figure (a) also illustrates the ability of MRI to image the hippocampal region clearly [E,F].

Figures (c) and (d) illustrate the extent of the left fornix damage (d[B]) relative to the intact right fornix (c[A]). The left-sided mammillary body damage can also be identified on these scans (d[D]) relative to the right (c[C]). (In figures c and d, the letters A and P in the top corners refer to anterior and posterior respectively.)

It is important to note that the left-hand side of each scan corresponds to the right-hand side of the brain.

19

When tested at two years, case 1 scored 43 and 45 on the word and face tests from the RMT, and, when tested at six months, case 2 scored 42 and 41 on the same tests. The patients' performances on the Logical Memory and the Paired Associate Learning Tests from the WMS–R fell below normal level to about the same extent as their performance on the RMT. At a delay of one hour, however, their performance was severely impaired. They were also slower than their control subjects to learn a list of eight words to a criterion of three perfect recalls, but even having reached this criterion, they could only recall a quarter of the words at 15 minutes delay, whereas their controls could recall all the words. This suggests that fornix lesions may have relatively little effect on either free recall or recognition at short delays, but that they cause an acceleration of forgetting such that the deficit becomes severe after a few minutes delay. In relation to the meta-analysis of Aggleton and Shaw (1996), this implies that, in patients with fornix lesions, free recall and forced choice recognition may be equally, and very mildly, impaired at short delays, but that free recall, at least, is severely impaired at longer delays because forgetting rate is accelerated for free recall. What happens to forced choice recognition after a longer delay in these patients is currently unknown. It is worth pointing out that monkeys who have received fornix lesions (and this probably also applies to selective hippocampal lesions) perform normally on delayed non-matching to sample tests at short delays in so far as these tasks tap object recognition memory (see Gaffan, 1992 for a discussion).

Hodges and Carpenter's (1991) two cases were also given tests of remote memory. Both patients performed within normal limits on tests about famous faces and famous events, and so revealed little evidence of temporally extensive retrograde amnesia for public information. Similarly, with personal memories, both patients produced as many memories as their controls to cues like flag, ship, and tree, and produced a similar proportion of memories from the previous five years as their controls. Although, immediately following the operation, case 1 had retrograde amnesia for the preceding year and case 2 for the preceding 14 months, both patients improved so that after several months their memory seemed normal except for the four weeks prior to surgery. These findings suggest that fornix lesions do not cause a temporally extensive retrograde amnesia although they may impair pre-morbid memories in a steeply temporally graded fashion.

We have given a series of neuropsychological tests to RM between 1994 and 1996 (four to six years after his surgery). The results of these tests are summarised in Table 2.1. His NART and WAIS–R scores give no indication that RM has suffered a decline in intelligence as a result of his colloid cyst and his surgery although his verbal IQ was marginally lower than his Performance IQ. RM's digit span was 8 and his visual memory span from the WMS–R was 5, which indicates that his short-term memory is preserved. Like the two patients of Hodges and Carpenter, the WMS–R also revealed that he

TABLE 2.1
Scores on Standardised Tests of Intelligence, Memory,
and Executive Functions

Test	RM	LA
GENERAL INTELLIGENCE TESTS		
WAIS–R: Full Scale IQ (Index)	88	86
Verbal IQ (Index)	85	88
Performance IQ (Index)	93	85
NART (Predicted Full Scale IQ)	86	105
MEMORY TESTS		
WMS–R: General (Index)	82	62
Verbal (Index)	76	62
Visual (Index)	100	90
Attn./Conc. (Index)	97	91
Delayed Recall (Index)	75	50
DOORS AND PEOPLE: Names (Percentile)	1	1
People (Percentile)	5	1
Doors (Percentile)	75–95	5
Shapes (Percentile)	75	1
WRMT: Words (Raw score)	43	33
Faces (Raw score)	42	29
FRONTAL TESTS		
Stroop (Percentile)	32	2
FAS (Raw score)	6.3	3.7
Cognitive Estimates (Raw score)	4	4

This shows RM's and LA's scores on standardised tests of
intelligence, memory, and executive functions. WAIS–R is the Wechsler
Adult Intelligence Scale–Revised; NART is the National Adult Reading
Test–Revised; WMS–S is the Wechsler Memory Scale–Revised; and the
FAS is the FAS Word Fluency Test.

is more impaired at verbal than visual memory. Although RM scores
considerably less than his similarly aged brother on the Visual Memory
Index, there is reason to believe that this index may be sensitive to verbal
memory (at which he is impaired) as well as visual (at which he may be
intact) (see Mayes, 1995). This impression is confirmed by RM's above
average performance on the visual recall and recognition tests of the Doors
and People Battery. This is consistent with the reports that his pre-morbid
memory was very good and suggests that his memory was better than that of at
least three-quarters of the population. We have no evidence that RM
initially had a deficit in visual memory that has subsequently recovered, as
was found with the patients of Hodges and Carpenter. His performance on the

RMT was very comparable to that of their patients as well and fell in the bottom quarter of the population. Given the apparent preservation of their visual memory, it is surprising that RM and case 2 of Hodges and Carpenter both perform marginally better on the verbal component of the RMT.

The Doors and People Test, which is currently the only instrument to allow direct comparison of impairment on verbal and visual recognition and free recall, gives a different impression. On this battery, whereas RM scored in the top quarter of the population on the visual forced choice recognition test, he performed in the bottom percent of the population on the verbal forced choice recognition test. His verbal recall score was in fact marginally better, lying in the bottom five percent of the population. It is interesting to compare RM's performance on this battery with that of his similarly aged brother, whose scores on the visual recall and recognition tests were very comparable, but who scored at the 50th and 75–90th percentiles on the verbal recognition and recall tests respectively. One could speculate that pre-morbidly RM was marginally better at verbal recall than verbal recognition, although another explanation of RM's severe verbal recognition deficit on the Doors and People battery is considered in the next paragraph.

RM's performance on tests of verbal free recall and recognition resembles that of Hodges and Carpenter's two patients in that he appears to be more impaired on the WMS–R Verbal Memory Index, which basically measures recall ability, than he is at the verbal component of the RMT, which taps forced choice recognition. However, it appears that this may not be true of other forced choice recognition tests. Whereas the RMT examines recognition memory for single words, the names test in the Doors and People battery examines recognition for first–second name combinations. It may therefore rely on memory for associations in a way that the RMT does not. In other words, immediately tested single item recognition may be relatively preserved after fornix lesions, but not immediately tested recognition memory for associations.

One feature of Hodges and Carpenter's two patients was that their delayed memory was more impaired than their memory when tested relatively immediately. This seemed to apply to RM to some extent, as his Delayed Memory Index showed somewhat more impairment than his General Memory Index, which relies on scores from memory tests given fairly immediately after study. To examine this issue further, we gave RM a test developed by Isaac (1994), which has been given to a large number of amnesics and matched control subjects. This test involves examining free recall and forced choice recognition for stories similar to those used in the Logical Memory subtest of the WMS–R. Free recall and recognition are tested at several filled delays (to prevent rehearsal) between 20 seconds and 10 minutes using different stories. The main twist to the procedure is that initial performance on free recall is matched at the 20 seconds delay between patients and control

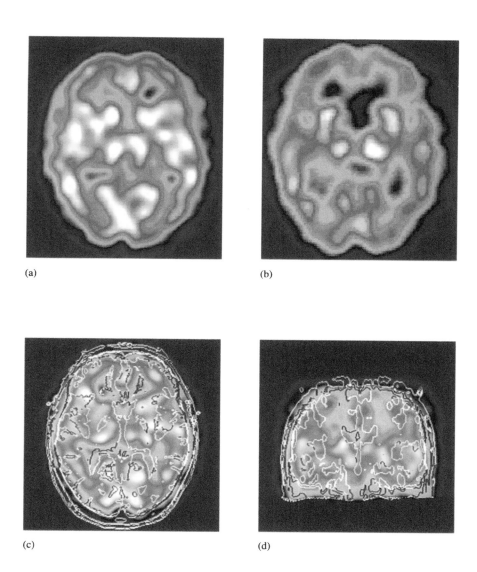

(a)

(b)

(c)

(d)

FIG. 2.1. Axial resting state SPECT scans of a normal healthy brain (a) and a damaged brain (b). High levels of rCBF are indicated by bright (yellow/white) areas while darker areas reflect reduced (red) or zero (grey/blue) blood flow. The scan of the damaged brain, therefore, indicates reduced rCBF in the posterior temporal region and almost no rCBF in the frontal lobes.

This figure also demonstrates SPECT–MRI co-registration of axial (c) and coronal (d) slices. This is discussed on pp. 12ff.

subjects by presenting the stories several times (nearly always five) to the amnesics. It was found that when the same procedure was followed for recognition, amnesics were also matched to their control subjects. We therefore concluded that at this delay free recall and recognition were equally impaired in the patients. After 10 minutes, however, although the amnesics had lost their recognition memory at a normal rate, their free recall of the stories had declined at a pathologically fast rate. At this delay, therefore, their free recall of the stories was more impaired than their recognition.

We have tested RM on this procedure twice at delays of 20 seconds and 10 minutes. The most striking finding was that his performance was completely normal on both free recall and recognition at the short delay even though he had only one exposure to the stories, which is the same as that given to normal people. We used a filled delay of 20 seconds because pilot work had indicated that when severe amnesics with normal short-term memory were tested at this delay after five presentations, they recalled practically nothing. We interpreted this to mean that there is a negligible contribution of short-term memory to free recall after a filled delay of 20 seconds. It would seem, therefore, that, in some respects, RM's memory is normal at delays sufficiently long for most amnesics to show recall and recognition deficits. Unlike normal people, he shows some loss of the ability both to free recall and to recognise the stories over 10 minutes. The effects were not strong, however, and RM's recognition at 10 minutes was, if anything, more impaired than his free recall. It remains unclear, therefore, whether RM's delayed forced choice recognition is any less impaired than his delayed free recall, at least for several such recognition tests.

In order to see how RM would perform when given a Yes/No recognition test matched for difficulty with a free recall test, we gave him Calev's (1984) task. This task involves a free recall test in which subjects see 24 words for four seconds each that are sequentially grouped into six categories of four words. Recall is allowed after subjects have been shown a three-digit number for five seconds and have then repeated it back. A recognition test is also given in which 40 unrelated words are given in the same way and recognition is tested in a Yes/No format with 40 foils, half of which rhyme with target words and half of which are semantically related to target words. Calev selected 24 critical words from the set of 40 targets such that normal subjects achieved the same number of recognition hits (15.1 out of 24) as they managed to free recall (15.6). On this task, we compared RM's scores with those of his brother. RM was able to free recall 14 words, and to recognise 22 out of the 24 critical words, in comparison with the 24 words recalled and 23 words recognised by his brother. RM did, however, show a high false alarm rate. He claimed to recognise 17 of the 40 foils, whereas his brother only falsely recognised five, and a group of 15 control subjects, who were matched to typical amnesics in age and intelligence, falsely recognised a mean of 7.7

foils. (These subjects actually free recalled 14.4 words and made 17.3 hits on the critical items.) Interestingly, we have also observed RM's high false alarm rate pattern on the Calev task in a patient with a relatively selective bilateral hippocampal lesion. Even though RM did show a false alarm rate that was nearly two standard deviations above that of the amnesic controls, his free recall and recognition performance lies close to that of the amnesic controls. This is true of RM's recognition memory sensitivity regardless of whether one corrects for false alarms using signal detection theory or threshold theory assumptions. Although it has to be admitted that RM's immediate Yes/No recognition and free recall are as good as matched control subjects, his memory may have been worsened under these conditions by his brain damage, as his memory was reported to be very good pre-morbidly. His brother's performance provides support for this possibility.

Whether the false alarm pattern represents an individual quirk or an effect of damage to the structures in the Papez circuit will require more patients with this lesion to be tested on the Calev task. If it is a systematic effect of the lesions, its cause will need to be identified. The simplest interpretation is that the patients have adopted a very liberal criterion for recognition. Alternatively, the patients may feel that they are remembering foil items to the same extent as they are remembering even the best-remembered target items. If the latter position were correct, then the patients would identify foil items as confidently as they identify targets.

RM does not show an entirely consistent pattern of deficit across all the tests of anterograde amnesia. This may be because his pre-morbid memory was well above average and has now only dropped slightly below normal levels. His brother's general memory and delayed memory indices, of 120 and 118 respectively, suggest that this may be so. Nevertheless, there is no strong evidence that his verbal free recall is more impaired than either his forced choice or his Yes/No recognition, and there is some evidence that his performance on all these tests may be relatively unimpaired at immediate test. His impairment is mild, but it may be that his immediate explicit memory is normal and that he then loses memory at an accelerated rate so that at longer delays his deficit becomes more dramatic. Anecdotal evidence indicates that at delays of more than an hour, his verbal memory deficits may become quite severe as was the case with the patients of Hodges and Carpenter.

Our tests of remote memory indicated that RM had some degree of retrograde amnesia, although the impairment was mild as was reported for the two patients of Hodges and Carpenter. There was little evidence of pre-morbid deficits in autobiographical memory, although RM was very poor at remembering post-morbid personal incidents. We asked RM's wife to recall certain incidents over the past few years that both RM and his brother had experienced. RM was not able to recall as much as his brother even for the pre-morbid memories. This indicates that he has a retrograde amnesia for personal events that may be steeply temporally graded like that of Hodges and Carpenter's patients. We tested his remote memory for public information with a test about famous events (Mayes et al., 1994). On this test, RM showed completely normal recognition of names of events from the 1980s and performed within a standard deviation of our amnesic controls on recognising names of events from the 1970s. The task required him to pick each correct name from three made-up ones. His ability to give the year of occurrence of the events that he recognised from these decades was, if anything, more accurate than that of the amnesic controls. He therefore resembles the patients of Hodges and Carpenter in showing little sign of retrograde amnesia for public information acquired years before the onset of his brain damage. It is, of course, quite possible that a more sensitive test of this kind would have shown a retrograde amnesia for public information with a very steep temporal gradient, matching the pattern displayed for his memory for personal events.

Finally, we examined RM's attentional functions using the Test of Everyday Attention (TEA). He had achieved an attention/concentration index within normal limits on the WMS–R, and the TEA failed to show any deficits on tests supposedly sensitive to the ability to concentrate in the presence of distraction. Although RM may have subtle attentional problems we suspect that these are of a kind likely to make a significant contribution to his memory deficits. The deficits are mild and specific to verbal material, but it is not clear that they affect recognition less than free recall. There is, however, a possibility that the memory deficit is greater after a delay. This would be consistent with fornix lesions causing a deficit in the storage of some or all aspects of fact and event information. This would not be inconsistent with the evidence that RM shows a mild retrograde amnesia that is steeply temporally graded.

Patient LA

The second patient, LA, was 49-year-old man who ran a hardware shop until he became ill in 1981. In the summer of that year, he suffered a spell of disorientation. In December of the same year, he suffered from what was probably an infarction that caused him suddenly to lose the sight of one eye, and to lose his senses of taste and smell. He is reported to have suffered a mild heart attack before 1981. The case notes are unclear, but over the next three years he became depressed and in 1986 he was admitted to a psychiatric hospital to have his depression treated. While he was in the hospital his memory problems were identified, but whether they began then, at the time of the incident in late 1981, or between the two, is unclear. So, all one can conclude with confidence is that between 1981 and 1986 he suffered one or more infarctions. His case notes are inadequate for unequivocal interpretation, but brief testing in 1986 led to the conclusion that he had verbal, but not non-verbal amnesia. However, two years later, he is reported to be globally amnesic. This suggests that somewhere between 1981 and 1986 (probably nearer 1986) he suffered a left-sided thalamic stroke, and that somewhere between 1986 and 1988 he suffered a right-sided thalamic stroke. After his discharge from the hospital, he has not been seriously depressed. Although he shows some degree of apathy and brief episodes of emotional lability, these may well result from his amnesia. There is no evidence that his condition has deteriorated, as his amnesia has remained at about the same level of severity since 1988. The only hint that he may have a continuing vascular problem occurred in 1989 when he awoke with a numb leg. He could walk on it, however, and the problem cleared within one day.

Our MRI scan of LA showed that he had suffered a bilateral infarction of the thalamus. The fornix, which runs very close to the anterior end of the thalamus, was intact and there was no evidence of focal damage to any of the other brain regions where lesions are believed to cause organic amnesia. Cortical atrophy was not greater than would be expected in a man in his early 60s. Although thalamic lesions are known sometimes to cause amnesia, the severity and qualitative features of the amnesia are very variable, particularly those relating to retrograde amnesia (see Butters & Stuss, 1989; Hodges, 1995), and the location of the critical damage is still not agreed. There are, however, strong grounds for thinking that the anterior and the dorsomedial nuclei are often involved, although their respective roles are uncertain. The mammillothalamic tract, which carries information from the mammillary bodies to the anterior nucleus, and the internal medullary lamina, which carries information from the amygdala to the dorsomedial nucleus, have also been implicated (see Mair, 1994). It has also been suggested by Mair (1994) that both the intralaminar and paralaminar non-specific thalamic nuclei may be involved.

LA's MRI scan is illustrated in Fig. 2.4. To see whether this would enable us to get a clearer picture of the anatomical causes of LA's severe amnesia, we used the thalamic atlases of Van Buren and Borke (1972) and Talairach and Tournoux (1988), and a procedure similar to that of Clarke et al. (1994). In our procedure, we aligned five of our MRI axial slices to five axial sections from the atlas that moved in 4mm steps from the bottom of the thalamus to the top. The scan had already shown that both lesions were just under 1cm in diameter and that the lesion on the left was inferior, medial, and anterior relative to the lesion on the right. On the lowest axial scan, there was no sign of a lesion on the right, but on the left there was a small area of damage encroaching on the anterior end of the dorsomedial nucleus and into the nucleus lateropolaris, which lies lateral and anterior to the dorsomedial nucleus. On the next scan up, the lesion on the right had begun in the anterior

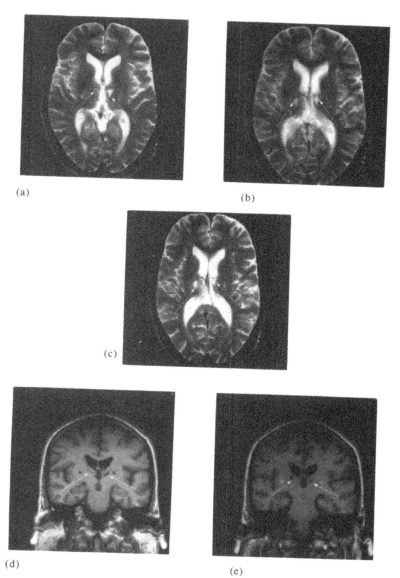

FIG. 2.4. Axial and coronal MRI scans illustrating the bilateral thalamic damage of LA. The three axials represent a low slice (a), a middle slice (b), and a high slice (c). Arrows [A], [C], and [E] illustrate the inferior, medial, and anterior position of the left infarct relative to the right [B], [D], and [F]).

The coronal slices (d) and (e) also illustrate the position and extent of the left ([G] and [J]) and right ([H] and [K]) lesions.

It is important to note that the left-hand side of each scan corresponds to the right-hand side of the brain.

27

dorsomedial nucleus and on the left had expanded to include not only the anterior dorsomedial thalamus and nucleus lateropolaris, but also the anterior nucleus, the mammillothalamic tract and the internal medullary lamina. On the third scan from the bottom, there was a small lesion still confined to the anterior dorsomedial thalamus on the right, whereas on the left there was a small amount of damage confined to the medial and posterior aspects of the dorsomedial thalamus. On the fourth scan, there was damage to the internal medullary lamina between the anterior nucleus and the nucleus lateropolaris, which probably extended into both these nuclei on the right, and, on the left, the lesion was reducing in size, but there was still some damage to the medial anterior thalamic nucleus. On the uppermost section, there was some damage to the nucleus lateropolaris on the right, while the left side was now clear.

Our neuropsychological tests revealed that LA's intelligence might have declined as a result either of ageing or of his infarct. His NART score indicated that he had an estimated pre-morbid IQ of 105 whereas his full scale IQ derived from his performance on the WAIS–R was 86 with Verbal and Performance IQs of 88 and 85 respectively. His performance on the Digit Span subtest yielded a scaled score of 6 and his forward span was only 5, which suggests that his verbal short-term memory is mildly impaired. His visual short-term memory span was 5, which is within normal limits for a man of his age. Our tests of his memory showed that he is severely amnesic. His Verbal and Visual Indices on the WMS–R of 62 and 90 suggest that he may have some sparing of visual memory. His scores on the Doors and People Test battery, however, give a different impression, as he scored at the first percentile level on all tests except the visual recognition task, on which he scored at the fifth percentile. Similarly, his performance on the RMT indicates that, if anything, his recognition memory for faces was slightly more impaired than his recognition memory for words. Consistent with his bilateral thalamic lesion, therefore, he appears to have an anterograde amnesia for verbal and non-verbal materials of more or less equivalent severity. Relative to RM, he has a much more severe anterograde amnesia, as is indicated by his WMS–R General Memory and Delayed Memory Indices, which are respectively 20 and 25 points lower than RM's.

LA's performance on our special purpose tests indicated the severity of his anterograde amnesia. On the forgetting rate task, he scored zero at a delay of 20 seconds on story recall after five study presentations, so we increased these to eight presentations at study. With these he was able to recall two gobbets of information at 20 seconds delay, but was unable to recall anything at two minutes delay. Under these conditions, he obtained a score of seven on recognition after a 20 second delay, but this had dropped to chance with a delay of two minutes. On the Calev test, his free recall score was only one word and this was the last word in the presentation and so was probably drawn from his short-term memory. On the Yes/No recognition test, he failed to identify any of the 80 test items whether they were targets or foils, so his score has to be returned as chance. One implication of these results is that not only is his explicit memory much more impaired than that of RM, but, unlike RM, he is severely impaired at both recognition and recall when these are tested without delay. His scores on Calev's test contrasted dramatically with those of RM, who scored in the normal range on both recall and recognition subtests.

LA's retrograde amnesia for personal events was very severe and there was little indication of sparing of the more remote events. In fact, the Autobiographical Memory Interview showed that he was unable to recall personal incidents from any period of his life. His retrograde amnesia for personal episodes is, therefore, severe and seems to be temporally ungraded. Examination of LA's performance on our famous events questionnaire (Mayes et al., 1994) indicates a striking pattern of performance. First, LA seems to show performance in the normal range with respect to his ability to identify the names of famous events from the 1970s, and his recognition of event names from the early 1980s before the onset of his amnesia is within one standard deviation of normal levels. His recognition for event names from the second half of the 1980s, after his amnesia developed, was, however, at least two standard deviations below the level of recognition shown by amnesic control subjects (Mayes et al., 1994). In comparison with his preserved recognition of pre-morbidly encountered public events, LA's recall of any details about the events of the early 1980s was severely impaired. For example, his ability to remember when the events of the early 1980s occurred was three standard deviations worse than that of the amnesic control subjects. In comparison, his memory for the temporal location of events from the 1970s was normal and from the later 1980s it was massively impaired (around nine standard deviations below the level shown by the amnesic controls).

There are three points worth making about these retrograde amnesia results. First, LA seems to show no evidence of having a temporally graded retrograde amnesia for personal episodes, but he does for public information knowledge about events. Second, he appears to show a similar pattern of deficit to the post-encephalitic amnesic, RFR, described by Warrington and McCarthy (1988), who showed a normal ability to recognise famous faces and names, despite very impaired ability to say anything about these recognised items. Like LA, this patient showed a very severe retrograde amnesia for personal and public information. Third, LA's impaired recognition for event names from the post-morbid part of the 1980s, and his inability to date the events that he could remember, indicate that additional factors must operate to produce his anterograde amnesia.

It is interesting to note that although both LA and RM perform within the normal range on the Cognitive Estimates Test (Shallice & Evans, 1978), they

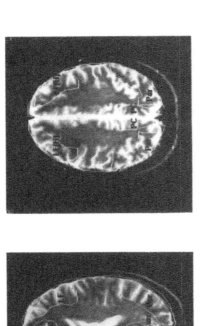
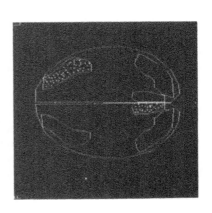

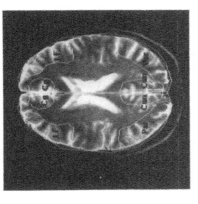
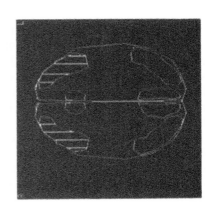

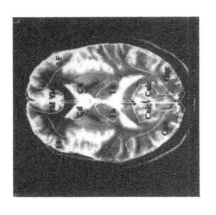
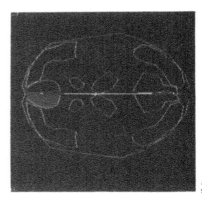

(a)

(b)

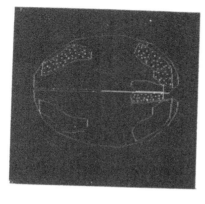

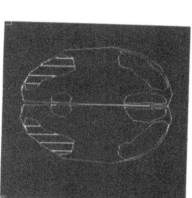

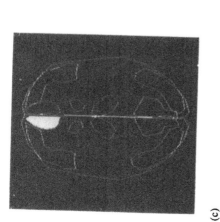

(c)

FIG. 2.5. Three axial MRI scans (a) illustrate the ROIs investigated. (See Fig. 2.2 for details and abbreviations.) The figure illustrates regions of blood flow change in RM (b) and LA (c). White and speckled areas indicate increased activation (z scores > 4 and between 2 and 4 respectively) while striped areas indicates decreased activation (z scores > 3). It is important to note that the left-hand side of each scan corresponds to the right-hand side of the brain.

31

seem very impaired on the FAS word fluency test. As both these tests supposedly tap planning ability and are meant to be sensitive to frontal lobe lesions, the latter impairment is important. Our structural MRI scans clearly show that there is no detectable frontal lobe damage in either patient. The ability to combine neuropsychology with neuroradiology here, therefore, enables us to demonstrate that the FAS is not selectively sensitive to frontal cortex damage. Whether the pattern of deficit on this test can be distinguished from deficits caused by frontal lobe planning problems remains to be determined.

LA, therefore, has impaired verbal short-term memory, a severe anterograde amnesia for both verbal and non-verbal information, and a severe retrograde amnesia with some interesting features. His impairment is more severe than that of RM. It may also not be qualitatively identical with respect to the verbal short-term memory deficit, the immediate onset of recognition and recall deficits in anterograde amnesia, and the pattern of retrograde amnesia. Our preferred hypothesis is that hippocampal circuit lesions, whether they are of the fornix or of the anterior thalamic nucleus, will produce a similar kind of memory deficit, which results from a failure to store complex associations such as those between items and their study context (but also the kinds of associations between two or more items that underlie semantic memory). The fact that LA's memory deficits may be slightly different in kind from RM's, in our view, is probably a result of his bilateral damage in the dorsomedial thalamic nucleus and the internal medullary lamina which leads to it from the amygdala. To establish this will, of course, require a group neuropsychological and neuroradiological study of many amnesic patients with thalamic lesions. If dorsomedial thalamic lesions do lead to this qualitative difference, this might be expected to show in the kind of SPECT study that we performed with the patients. It is unclear whether this study will show why LA has a more severe memory deficit.

COMPARISON OF RM AND LA ON THE SPECT STUDY

Both patients to varying degrees conformed to the amnesic group difference from the controls matched to them on recall level. That is, they showed less right lateral frontal and more left lateral frontal activation than did the control subjects. Both RM and LA showed this trend, but they differed with respect to the activation they showed in the right ventromedial frontal cortex when their activation levels were converted to z scores based on the control group's means and standard deviations. This is illustrated in Fig. 2.5. RM's activation in this region was several z score units lower than LA's. This frontal region is known to receive projections from both the anterior thalamus (and hence indirectly the hippocampus) and the dorsomedial thalamus (and hence indirectly the amygdala). These projections may well be disrupted in the case of LA, as both these nuclei are damaged on the right side of his brain, but RM has no right-sided structural damage. The reduced level of activation shown by RM cannot be a simple consequence of his structural damage, and may perhaps indicate that the two patients are doing the task in a distinct way, with LA showing an abnormal heightening of activation relative to the normal control group.

The patients also differed in the left parietal lobe activation that they showed, with LA demonstrating more activation. This is interesting, but at present we are unable to explain it anatomically or functionally because, although our study indicates that parietal activation results from successful retrieval, it does not indicate what aspect(s) of successful retrieval are responsible for the activation. Others of the patients showed markedly different precuneus activation and this probably reflects the different extent to which they used imagery in retrieval. As with the ventromedial frontal cortex, it could be argued that LA, who has more cortical projection systems damaged on both left and right sides of the brain, could be showing more activation in both the left parietal and right ventromedial frontal cortex because the lesioned nuclei normally exert an inhibitory effect on their cortical targets. We still need to determine whether LA shows more widespread cortical effects than does RM, which may underlie his more serious memory problems.

CONCLUSION

In this chapter, we have made the argument that advances in our understanding of amnesia are going to depend increasingly on combining detailed and hypothesis-driven testing of patients with selective brain lesions with careful structural and functional neuroradiological procedures. The neuroradiological techniques should enable the investigator to identify the structural damage in life that is present around the time that the neuropsychological testing is administered, and also to examine what the functional effects of this structural damage are both while in a resting state and when engaging the processing that has been compromised.

ACKNOWLEDGEMENTS

All the neuroradiological work described in this chapter was carried out at the Institute of Neurological Sciences, Glasgow under the supervision of Dr. Donald Hadley and Dr. David Wyper.

REFERENCES

Aggleton, J.P., & Shaw, C. (1996). Amnesia and recognition memory: A re-analysis of psychometric data. *Neuropsychologia, 34*, 51–62.

Bandettini, P.A., Kwong, K.K., Davis, T.L., Iiang, A., Baker, I.R., Belliveau, I.W., Weiskoff, R.M., & Rosen, B.R. (1995). FMRI demonstrates sustained blood oxygenation and flow enhancement during extended duration visual and motor cortex activation. *Society for Neuroscience, 21*, 1209.

Butters, N., & Stuss, D.T. (1989). Diencephalic amnesia. In L. Squire & G. Gainotti (Eds.), *Handbook of neuropsychology*, Vol. 3. Amsterdam: Elsevier.

Calev, A. (1984). Recall and recognition in chronic nondemented schizophrenics. *Journal of Abnormal Psychology, 93*, 172–177.

Clarke, S., Assal, G., Bogousslavsky, J., Regli, F., Townsend, D.W., Leenders, K.L., & Blecic, S. (1994). Pure amnesia after unilateral left polar thalamic infarct: Topographic and sequential neuropsychological and metabolic (PET) correlations. *Journal of Neurology, Neurosurgery and Psychiatry, 57*, 27–34.

Fletcher, C., Frith, C.D., Baker, S.C., Shallice, T., Frackowiak, R.S.J., & Dolan, R.J. (1995). The mind's eye precuneus activation in memory-related imagery. *Neuroimage, 2*, 195–200.

Gaffan, D. (1992). The role of the hippocampus–fornix–mammillary system in episodic memory. In L.R. Squire & N. Butters (Eds.), *Neuropsychology of memory*, 2nd edn. New York: Guilford Press.

Grady, C.L., McIntosh, A.R., Horwitz, B., Maisog, J.M., Ungerleider, L.G., Mentis, M.J., Pietrini, P., Schapiro, M.B., & Haxby, J.V. (1995). Age-related reductions in human recognition memory due to impaired encoding. *Science, 269*, 218–221.

Hodges J. (1995). Retrograde amnesia. In A.D. Baddeley, B.A. Wilson & F.N. Watts (Eds.), *Handbook of memory disorders*. Chichester: John Wiley.

Hodges, J.R., & Carpenter, K. (1991). Anterograde amnesia with fornix damage following removal of third ventricle colloid cyst. *Journal of Neurology, Neurosurgery and Psychiatry, 54*, 633–638.

Isaac, C. (1994). *Rate of forgetting of verbal material in amnesia*. Unpublished PhD Dissertation, Manchester University, UK.

Kapur, S., Craik, F.I.M., Tulving, E., Wilson, A.A., Houle, S., & Brown, G.M. (1994). Neuroanatomical correlates of encoding in episodic memory: Levels of processing effect. *Proceedings of the National Academy of Sciences*, USA, *91*, 2008–2011.

Lencz, T., McCarthy, G., Bronen, R.A., Scott, T.M., Inserni, J.A., Sass, K.J., Novelly, R.A., Kim, J.H., & Spencer, D.D. (1992). Quantitative magnetic resonance imaging in temporal lobe epilepsy: Relationship to neuropathology and neuropsychological function. *Annals of Neurology, 31*, 629–637.

Levasseur, M., Baron, J.C., Sette, G., Legault-Demare, F., Pappata, S., Mauguiere, F., Benott, N., Dinh, S.T., Degos, J.D., Laplane, D., & Mazoyer, B. (1992). Brain energy metabolism in bilateral paramedian thalamic infarcts. *Brain, 115*, 795–807.

Mair, R.G. (1994). On the role of thalamic pathology in diencephalic amnesia. *Reviews in the Neurosciences, 5*, 105–140.

Mayes, A.R. (1988). *Human Organic Memory Disorders*. Cambridge: Cambridge University Press.

Mayes, A.R. (1995). The assessment of memory disorders. In A.D. Baddeley, B.A. Wilson & F.N. Watts (Eds.), *Handbook of memory disorders*. Chichester: Wiley.

Mayes, A.R., Downes, J.J., MacDonald, C., Poole, V., Rooke, S., Sagar, H.J., & Meudell, P.R. (1994). Two tests for assessing remote public knowledge: A tool for assessing retrograde amnesia. *Memory, 2*, 183–210.

Mayes, A.R., Meudell, P.R., Mann, D., & Pickering, A.D. (1988). Location of lesions in Korsakoff's syndrome: Neuropsychological and neuropathological data on two patients. *Cortex, 24*, 1–22.

Schacter, D.L., Reiman, E., Uecker, A., Polster, M.R., Yung, L.S., & Cooper, L.A. (1995). Brain regions associated with retrieval of structurally coherent visual information. *Nature, 376*, 537–540.

Shallice, T., & Evans, M.E. (1978). The involvement of the frontal lobes in cognitive estimation. *Cortex, 14*, 294–303.

Shallice, T., Fletcher, P., Frith, C.D., Grasby, P., Frackowiak, R.S.J., & Dolan, R.J. (1994). Brain regions associated with acquisition and retrieval of verbal episodic memory. *Nature, 328*, 633–635.

Soininen, H.S., Partanen, K., Pitkanen, A., Vainio, P., Hanninen, T., Hallikainen, M., Koivisto, K., & Riekkinen, P.J. (1994). Volumetric MRI analysis of the amygdala and the hippocampus in subjects with age-associated memory impairment: Correlation to visual and verbal memory. *Neurology, 44*, 1660–1668.

Talairach, J., & Tournoux, P. (1988). Co-planar stereotaxic atlas of the human brain. New York: Thieme Medical Publishers.

Tulving, E., Kapur, S., Markowitsch, H.J., Craik, F.I.M., Habib, R., & Houle, S. (1994). Neuroanatomical correlates of retrieval in episodic memory: Auditory sentence recognition. *Proceedings of the National Academy of Sciences, USA, 91*, 2012–2015.

Ungerleider, L.G. (1995). Functional brain imaging studies of cortical mechanisms of memory. *Science, 270*, 769–775.

Van Buren, J.M., & Borke, R.C. (1972). *Variations and connections of the human thalamus. 1. The nuclei and cerebral connections of the human thalamus.* Berlin: Springer Verlag.

Victor, M., Adams, R.D., & Collins, G.H. (1989). *The Wernicke–Korsakoff Syndrome and related neurological disorders due to alcoholism and malnutrition.* 2nd edn. Philadelphia: F.A. Davis Company.

Warrington, E.K., & McCarthy, R.A. (1988). The fractionation of retrograde amnesia. *Brain and Cognition, 7*, 184–200.

3 Autobiographical Amnesia and Temporal Lobe Pathology

Narinder Kapur
*Wessex Neurological Centre, Southampton, UK
and Department of Psychology, University of Southampton, UK*

INTRODUCTION

Autobiographical amnesia has in recent years become recognised as an important feature of memory disorder in neurological patients (Conway, Rubin, Spinnler, & Wagenaar, 1992; Dall'Ora, Della Sala, & Spinnler, 1989; Kapur, 1993). Some patients may display autobiographical memory loss as part of a focal retrograde amnesia (Goldberg et al., 1981; Kapur et al., 1992), while in others it may be a feature of a global amnesic condition (Dalla Barba, Cipolotti, & Denes, 1990; Hodges & McCarthy, 1993). Apart from these well-described cases of marked memory disorder, the occurrence of autobiographical memory symptoms as a more general clinical feature in routine neuropsychological practice has hitherto been somewhat ignored and possibly underestimated. Where loss of past memories occurs to a significant degree, it may have a major impact on the everyday adjustment of the patient and his/her family. Shared autobiographical memories, shared facts about the world, etc. may no longer be available to the patient and his/her family, and this may therefore have a disruptive effect on the relationships and the well-being of the patient and also of his/her carers.

There is little hard evidence relating to the pathophysiological or anatomical mechanisms underlying autobiographical amnesia as such, but the more general memory loss associated with retrograde amnesia has attracted speculation from clinicians and researchers. At the beginning of the century, Cowles (1900) reviewed earlier reports of retrograde amnesia associated with

37

epilepsy, and he presented his own case of retrograde amnesia associated with a possible epileptic seizure. It is worth noting that Alzheimer (quoted in Cowles, 1900), before studying the primary degenerative dementia that was to make him so renowned, wrote about retrograde amnesia associated with epilepsy. One of Alzheimer's patients had a retrograde amnesia of over a year following an epileptic seizure, although this seemed to have recovered in the subsequent weeks. Alzheimer remarked that retrograde amnesia in some cases of epilepsy may cover the whole of the preceding life.

Over 30 years ago, the neurologist Sir Charles Symonds (1962, p.3) alluded to the possibility that temporal lobe mechanisms may be critical to the presence and severity of retrograde amnesia

> I believe, therefore, we must accept the probability that the ordinary retrograde amnesia of concussion is produced by bilateral and symmetrical injury to the nerve-fibres in the cerebral hemispheres, which need not be situated in the temporal lobes. But there are cases in which the retrograde amnesia has unusual features, and these variants may represent selective temporal lobe damage.

There is now further evidence from several investigations that the severe autobiographical memory loss found in some cases of retrograde amnesia may be particularly associated with temporal lobe damage (e.g. De Renzi & Lucchelli, 1993; Markowitsch et al., 1993; O'Connor et al., 1992). There is also some tentative evidence that left temporal lobe lesions are more likely than right temporal lobe lesions to result in autobiographical memory impairment (Barr, Goldberg, Wasserstein, & Novelly, 1990; Yoneda, Yamadori, Mori, & Yamashita, 1992).

In this chapter, I examine the occurrence of autobiographical memory symptoms in a number of patients where it was one of the major presenting clinical features. In none of these patients was there a classical amnesic syndrome. Three types of conditions are presented where symptoms of autobiographical memory loss were a major feature of the patient's clinical profile—(A) Temporal Lobe Epilepsy, (B) Vertebrobasilar Insufficiency, and (C) Severe Head Injury. Six case reports are described. Autobiographical memory loss is, by its very nature, relatively unique to each individual and rather difficult to quantify in a standardised manner. Thus, some of these case studies mainly comprise qualitative reports of memory loss, either recounted by the patient or by a close relative.

(A) TEMPORAL LOBE EPILEPSY

Case 1

PO, a right-handed man (d.o.b. 19 February 1922) who once worked as a high-ranking civil servant, first presented in November 1984 to his company doctor at the age of 62. He complained that in the previous month he had woken up and did not know what he was meant to be doing that day, nor did he know how to get to work. He did not have any memory for the previous day. This period of confusion cleared up after an hour. The only other symptom that PO recounted was attacks of misty vision while sitting at his desk, these lasting for about 10 minutes. Physical examination at that time did not show any abnormality.

One month later, he went to his general practitioner indicating that he had suffered two or three further similar episodes of memory loss, each lasting about an hour, and also mentioned the occurrence of shorter periods of blurred vision and slurred speech. Physical examination was again unremarkable.

PO was seen by a consultant neurologist in February 1985. When describing the episode of memory loss in October, he was able to remember that he got dressed and read a newspaper in the morning. On this occasion, he recounted a similar episode six weeks later (i.e. late November/early December). In the morning, he awoke in a confused state, not knowing what day it was. Later in the morning, his wife found him in his car in the garage with the engine running. He was in a "confused" state and did not know what he was meant to be doing that day. It also appears that later in the morning he lost consciousness for a short period of time. When he became conscious again he did not know where he lived, but by midday he had recovered from his "confusional" state. There was no specific evidence of any epileptic fit having occurred. On the occasion of this appointment, PO reported weekly episodes of blurred vision, usually in the middle of the morning while he was at his desk. In addition to his vision being blurred, he would see a 'V'-shaped pattern with spots in front of his eyes, and he would be partly confused at this point in time. Afterwards he would have a slight headache and be somewhat sleepy. He also reported occasional episodes of slurred speech, staggering—usually on getting up in the mornings—and two occasions of abnormal taste, a combination of acetone and a fatty taste, lasting once for a few days and once for a whole week. PO also complained of more general deterioration in his memory functioning, such that it was affecting his performance at work. Physical examination did not reveal anything of note. It was thought that some of his symptoms reflected vertebrobasilar insufficiency and/or temporal lobe abnormality.

In March 1985, PO again presented to his general practitioner, complaining that for the last 4–6 weeks he had developed a progressive loss of taste and smell, and also noted a strange taste sensation ("sweet/sickly") in his mouth. In May 1985 PO reported that his memory had deteriorated to the extent that he could not remember the previous days' events at work—e.g. when he looked at letters that he had recently written he had no recollection that he had in fact written them. He also complained of some emotional instability and the feeling that people's faces sometimes appeared "odd" to him, as if his visual perception was impaired.

A CT scan around this time was normal. EEG investigations showed some bitemporal abnormality, more marked in the left temporal lobe. On 5 June 1985 PO was seen for neuropsychological assessment. His wife reported that, in addition to the amnesic episodes, PO could not remember their moving house in September 1984 nor their moving house in January 1981, and that on one occasion he did not remember the place where they had lived for 12 years. She reported that most mornings PO did not appear to know what day it was, that he had difficulty in knowing the directions to get to work, and that his memory for the previous eight months was almost "blank". She thought that his "everyday" memory was good for information that was minutes or a few hours old, but that it was very poor for events that occurred more than 1–2 days previously.

In June 1985, when PO was again seen by a consultant neurologist, he reported the occurrence of two further amnesic episodes. On 2 July 1985 PO had an epileptic fit, which occurred during the night, and had a further nocturnal fit one week later. Since that time, he has been successfully treated with anti-convulsant medication, and apart from one minor fit in February 1986, he has not had any further recurrence either of major epileptic attacks or of his more frequent, transient "confusional" states. Repeat CT scanning and EEG examinations did not show any changes in the findings that had been obtained from the earlier investigations.

PO was seen for more detailed neuropsychological investigations between April 1988 and June 1990. His symptoms and pattern of cognitive performance differed little over this time period. At the time of this assessment, he was taking Tegretol to control his epilepsy. On this occasion, he thought that his "everyday" memory was only mildly impaired. He was aware of a "gap" in his memory stretching back around 10 years, such that he had difficulty in visualising places or people that had been familiar in this period. He thought that this aspect of his memory loss had shown some improvement over the past two years since he started taking anti-convulsant medication. He reported that his sense of taste and smell had now recovered to normal. He did not remember seeing me before in 1985 nor coming to this hospital to undergo psychological testing. He had resumed driving for the past six months, and commented that he usually needed a map to get around to places that had generally been familiar to him in the past.

Autobiographical Memory Loss. His wife reported that PO's everyday memory was relatively good for information up to a day or so previously, but was impaired for information from longer ago than this. Thus, on one occasion a television film which had been shown at Xmas (about four months previously), and which both PO and his wife had watched, had recently been repeated, but PO had no recollection of having seen it before. Similarly, on the way to the hospital he did not remember that he had been in the area a few months earlier. She observed that PO no longer had any transient "confusional" episodes either in the morning or during the day. She commented that when they travelled somewhere in the locality he usually did not have any "visual idea" of where he was going, and that this applied both to familiar or unfamiliar places. She considered that his autobiographical memory loss stretched as far back as the early 1960s. She did not think he was suffering from any degree of depression or other psychiatric illness.

PO's autobiographical memory was formally assessed by conducting an in-depth interview with his wife regarding events/information over the past 50 years and then asking PO about the same items. A range of topics were covered, including schooling, occupations, places of residence, health, children, and visits abroad.

PO could accurately remember his secondary schooling. Because his father was in the armed forces, he went to four separate secondary schools. He could recall three of these spontaneously, and when cued with regard to the fourth he did remember having attended there. He was able to visualise the schools and also the schoolmasters. He remembered serving in the Far East during World War II, being posted in Malta after the war, and attending a Scientific Civil Service College in the early 1950s.

He could remember his marriage, where he got married, and the name of his best man. He could not, however, picture in his mind the church in which he got married, and he did not think he would recognise it if it was before him. He remembered having a short honeymoon in England; but could not recall the name of the town where they had spent this time, nor could he picture in his mind any of the honeymoon. Because he was working for the army or Ministry of Defence from the early 1950s onwards, he made various changes of residence. He was able to recount these accurately, and was also able to indicate the years and places of birth in respect of three of his children who were born in 1955, 1957, and 1959. His memory for changes of residence during the 1960s was normal, and he was also able to recall the years when his father and his father-in-law died (in 1972 and 1962). However, he did not recall that his son had an operation for tonsillectomy in 1968.

He was able to indicate that his father died in 1972 and could clearly describe the situation in which he was told of his father's death. He could remember the journey to the funeral, but could not visualise the funeral itself. He could recall that his mother died in the early 1970s, a few years after his father, but he could not picture the day she died as he could in the case of his father. He could not remember his son having an operation for appendicitis in 1975. He could remember the place where he lived in the 1970s, but could not give an accurate description of the design of the rooms, nor could he recall that he had had the front windows of his house replaced. He could not recall his 25th wedding anniversary in 1979, nor remember the party that had been held for this occasion. He was able to recall receiving hospital treatment for a back problem, but he could not picture the ward or any of the staff.

He could not recall his daughter's wedding in 1980 nor his son's wedding in 1981. Even when he was shown photographs of these occasions, these did not evoke any sense of familiarity for him. He could not recollect his transfer of residence in 1981, nor could he give a detailed account of the design of the house in which he lived for the following three years. He did not recall receiving several bee stings in 1981—these were quite significant events (he kept a bee hive at his home around that time), as he reacted adversely to the sting on each occasion, and in one instance he required hospital treatment. He could recall a trip to the United States in 1982, but his wife indicated that his memory for this event had only recently returned after they had gone over the event many times. He could not remember a transfer of residence in October 1984.

In summary, PO has fairly marked autobiographical memory loss for events covering approximately 10 years prior to the onset of his illness in 1984, mainly covering items from the 1970s and early 1980s. Memory for events from the 1940s through to the 1960s appears relatively normal, with only one or two isolated episodes that are not remembered. The only formal indication that some aspects of PO's autobiographical memory prior to the 1960s might not be completely intact came from a test given in June 1990, when he and his wife were separately asked to describe the exterior and interior of the various dwellings in which they had lived prior to PO's illness. PO could offer little in the way of detailed description of the houses in which he had lived, even going back to the home in which he had grown up, whereas his wife was able to give a much clearer and more detailed verbal sketch of each dwelling.

Neuropsychological Assessment.   PO was administered all 11 subtests of the Wechsler Adult Intelligence Scale–Revised (Wechsler, 1981). His IQ scores are indicated in Table 3.1, and show a uniformly above-average level of performance. On a card sorting task (Nelson, 1982), he was only able to achieve two categories (shape and number), but after the task he simply indicated that he did not think of colour (he was able to name the colours accurately), and on the more sensitive measure of proportion of perseverative errors his score (17%) was much lower than the recommended cut-off point of 50% errors which is considered suggestive of frontal lobe dysfunction. On verbal memory testing, his immediate and delayed (30min) recall of a short story was unimpaired, with immediate and delayed scores falling between the 75th and 90th percentiles (Coughlan & Hollows, 1985). His verbal

TABLE 3.1.
PO's WAIS–R IQ Test Scores

	Verbal IQ	Performance IQ	Full Scale IQ	Subtest Scores (Age-scaled)
WAIS-R	119	124	122	Information–15
				Digit Span–12
				Vocabulary–4
				Arithmetic–13
				Comprehension–12
				Similarities–13
				Picture Completion–16
				Picture Arrangement–13
				Block Design–14
				Object Assembly–12
				Digit Symbol–14

recognition memory performance (Warrington, 1984) was unimpaired (45/ 50). On a corresponding faces recognition memory task, he obtained a similar unimpaired score (47/50). On a design learning task (Coughlan & Hollows, 1985), his performance reflected a mild impairment—on the three learning components of this task his scores were at the 10th, 25th, and 75th percentiles, and for none of his scores was his performance below the recommended cut-off of two standard deviations below the mean. PO was also administered the Wechsler Memory Scale–Revised (Wechsler, 1987). As can be seen in Table 3.2, he performed at an average or above-average level on the various index scores.

TEMPORAL LOBE EPILEPSY SECONDARY TO SYSTEMIC LUPUS ERYTHEMATOSIS

Case 2

RS, a right-handed travel agent (d.o.b. 15 December 1942), suffered two episodes of deep vein thrombosis in 1982. In November 1985 he had an episode of loss of consciousness, although it was uncertain as to whether this represented an epileptic seizure. This was followed one year later by a definite seizure, after which he commenced taking anti-convulsant medication. He reported that since that time he had experienced one or two episodes in which he felt vague and slightly removed from what was going on around him. In January 1989 he suffered a minor fit lasting 30 seconds during which he looked glazed and distant, and repeated the same phrase several times.

TABLE 3.2.
PO's Memory Test Scores

Test	Raw Score	Statistic Score
Revised Wechsler		
Memory Scale		
General Memory		110
Verbal Memory		113
Visual Memory		105
Attention/Concentration		115
Delayed Recall		118
Logical Memory (Immediate)		87 percentile
Logical Memory (Delayed)		81 percentile
Visual Reproduction (Immediate)		96 percentile
Visual Reproduction (Delayed)		98 percentile
Recognition Memory Test		
Word recognition	45/50	11 (scaled-score)
Faces recognition	47/50	13 (scaled-score)
Adult Memory and Information		
Processing Battery		
Story recall		
Immediate recall	28/56	75–90 percentile
Delayed (30min) recall	28/56	75–90 percentile
Word-list learning		
List one	51	50–75 percentile
List two	5	50 percentile
Delayed recall		
List one	6	10-25 percentile
Complex figure recall		
Immediate recall	70/76	>90 percentile
Delayed (30min) recall	66/76	75–90 percentile
Design learning		
Design one	17/45	10 percentile
Design two	4/9	25 percentile
Delayed recall		
Design one	5/9	75 percentile

A magnetic resonance scan (MR) carried out in December 1988 showed a few minor ischaemic lesions, two of which were periventricular. A further MR scan in April 1990 showed multiple areas of high signal in the white matter of both cerebral hemispheres, the largest of these being adjacent to the trigone of the left lateral ventricle. Further small lesions were present in the brain stem and clustered around the fourth ventricle. This lesion profile was confirmed in a more recent scan carried out in March 1992. An EEG carried out in 1992 showed a possible left temporal lobe abnormality, although there was also thought to be considerable artefact in this recording.

Autobiographical Memory Loss. RS presented in 1988 with complaints of autobiographical memory difficulties that were more prominent for past events than for more current everyday situations. He indicated that his memory for personal past events occurring over the past 10 years was rather poor. He first became aware of memory difficulties for past events around two years previously. Examples of such memory difficulties included the following: he indicated that he went on a two-week holiday in Gambia about a year previously, but now had no memory for this; two years previously he went to Cairo for two weeks, and his only remaining memory for this holiday was of the boat, on which he was cruising, being stuck in a lock (he thought that this particular memory only remained because of a photograph of the event which he has retained). RS indicated that his memory for events was usually intact for a few weeks after the episode, but after this his memory for the event would gradually fade.

In addition to memory loss for specific events such as holidays, he also reported difficulty in recalling routes that he once knew well—e.g. 10–12 years previously he used to work in London as a taxi dispatcher, and knew his way around the city very well, but now had difficulty in finding his way around London. In addition, up to three years previously he used to know a particular tourist route around Europe very well (this covered World War II battlefield sites), having driven the tourist coach on a number of occasions, but when he went on this trip the previous year he had great difficulty in recalling the route. By contrast, RS considered that his memory in everyday situations was less noticeably impaired. This latter memory difficulty appeared to be present for the past 6–7 years, with some deterioration over that time; thus, he usually wrote down things that he had to remember. He did not admit to any difficulty in recognising familiar faces, although he did admit to some difficulty in retrieving their names. He also reported occasional naming difficulty, especially with items such as brand names.

RS's partner thought that his long-term (several months) memory for material such as faces was quite poor but that his memory for more recent and everyday material—e.g. remembering to do things—was either intact or only mildly impaired.

RS's autobiographical memory was assessed by means of a structured interview covering past personal events, using procedures similar to those described elsewhere. The particular items selected for this interview were based on an initial interview with RS's partner, and covered the following areas: educational experience, hospital treatments, holidays, occupational history, houses in which he had lived, births and deaths in his family, his present (non-marital) relationship, and his two earlier marriages.

On the basis of this interview with RS, there was some memory loss for several events that occurred in the 6–12 month period prior to November 1985. Thus, RS did not have any clear recollection of the birth of his child in

June 1985, nor of a holiday he had in Thailand and Hong Kong in November 1984.

At a follow-up assessment in March 1990, RS continued to have major memory loss for significant personal past events. Thus, he could not picture his first wedding in the early 1960s nor his second marriage in the early 1970s. A year earlier (February 1991), he had visited New Zealand and Hong Kong. While he could recall parts of the New Zealand visit, he had only a very vague recollection of the trip to Hong Kong, which lasted four days, and he could not recall two previous visits he had made to Hong Kong in the 1970s. On this occasion, we did administer the Autobiographical Memory Interview (Kopelman, Wilson, & Baddeley, 1990), which had become available in the intervening years. RS performed normally on personal semantic items, but his scores were "probably abnormal" for autobiographical incidents recalled from his childhood (score = 4/9), and "borderline" for events recalled from his early adult life (5/9). More recent incidents were recalled normally (7/9). These data complement those from our more open-ended interview with RS and his partner, although it is our experience that the more structured and more focused questions in the Autobiographical Memory Interview may sometimes underestimate the true extent of retrograde amnesia that is present.

Neuropsychological Assessment. Most of the following procedures were carried out in early 1989. On general cognitive tasks, RS did not show any major deficits. On the Wechsler Adult Intelligence Scale–Revised (Wechsler, 1981), he obtained a Verbal IQ of 103, a Performance IQ of 93, and a Full Scale IQ of 99. On an adult reading test (Nelson, 1982), his score was equivalent to an IQ of 113—as this reading test was validated on the Wechsler Adult Intelligence Scale rather than Wechsler Adult Intelligence Scale–Revised, the real drop in IQ test scores is probably fairly mild. His age-scaled scores on various WAIS–R subtests were generally within normal limits: Information = 11, Arithmetic = 13, Similarities = 10, Picture Arrangement = 9, Block Design = 10, Digit Symbol = 10. On the modified Wisconsin Card Sorting Test (Nelson, 1976), although he only obtained three categories, few of his errors were of a perseverative nature, and from his own verbal report after the task he appeared to be looking for more complex strategies than the correct ones. He performed within normal limits on a verbal fluency test and could name 20 words beginning with the letter "s" in 90 seconds.

Anterograde memory was assessed using a range of memory tests. His performance on the Revised Wechsler Memory Scale (Wechsler, 1987) showed patchy impairment. He had a Verbal Memory Quotient of 118, a Visual Memory Quotient of 81, a General Memory Quotient of 104, a Delayed Recall Quotient of 88, and an Attention/Concentration Quotient of 102. More informative data on RS's memory functioning comes from his subtest scores—the subtests where he showed impairment were Visual Reproduction, immediate and delayed, and Visual Paired-Associate learning (9/18). On other subtests, he performed normally. On a design learning and a word-list learning test (Coughlan & Hollows, 1985), he showed moderately impaired performance on only one of the three measures—delayed recall after an interference trial for the verbal memory task, and learning performance over five trials for the nonverbal memory task. On a words and a faces recognition memory test (Warrington, 1984), he performed at a low average level on both tests (42/50 for words, 41/50 for faces).

(B) VERTEBROBASILAR INSUFFICIENCY

Case 3

JE, a 63-year-old right-handed retired architect (d.o.b 16 August 1926) presented in 1990 and 1991 with a history of tremor suggestive of the presence of Parkinson's Disease, and with symptoms to suggest the presence of vertebrobasilar insufficiency—episodes of dizzy spells/unsteadiness and double vision. An MR scan was normal. Both he and his wife reported that his everyday "shorter-term" memory was intact, but that he suffered major memory loss for recent events that he had experienced.

Autobiographical Memory Loss. In September 1990, his wife noted that they had taken a trip to Australia the year before, and vast chunks of that holiday had disappeared from his memory. During the summer of 1990, they had gone on a holiday to Ireland and he had also forgotten much of that holiday. Occasionally, such autobiographical memory loss resulted in more focal verbal memory symptoms: for example, he sat on several committees, and he made suggestions that people would have to remind him that he had already made in the past. When seen in October 1990, he reported that when shown photographs of a holiday in Lancashire on which he went with some friends, he did not have any recollection of the holiday or of particular events such as a trip on a barge. When he watched video films of family events that he had taken with his camcorder, these appeared totally new to him. He also confessed to difficulty in finding his way around familiar places such as towns that he knew well.

Neither he nor his wife reported any episodes of transient global amnesia (TGA), but his wife did point to two episodes of transient "confusion". One was during a holiday in Skye seven years before. It began sometime in the morning and lasted around an hour, during which JE did not know where he was, what he was doing there, or how he got there. There was, however, no repetitive questioning as one finds in TGA. There subsequently remained a gap in his memory for this period. A further episode occurred four years previously, when he went to Salisbury cathedral. The next morning, he was rather confused about the previous day and did not have any clear memory for the trip the day before. He subsequently had a complete memory loss for this visit to Salisbury.

On the Autobiographical Memory Interview (Kopelman et al., 1990), he had perfect performance on the Personal Semantic items, obtaining maximum scores on each section. For Autobiographical Incidents, his scores for Childhood and Recent Life were normal (9 and 8 respectively), but his score of 6 for Early Adult Life was "borderline".

Neuropsychological Assessment.   JE was administered six subtests of the Wechsler Adult Intelligence Scale–Revised (Wechsler, 1981). He obtained a Verbal IQ of 117, a Performance IQ of 101, and a Full Scale IQ of 111. On a card sorting task (Nelson, 1982), he had a perfect score. On the Wechsler Memory Scale–Revised (Wechsler, 1987), he had Visual and Verbal Memory Quotients of 106 and 114 respectively, and a Delayed Memory Quotient of 119. He did not show any impairment of the words or faces versions of the Recognition Memory Test (Warrington, 1984).

(C) SEVERE HEAD INJURY

Although the residual autobiographical amnesia in the following case is rather patchy and primarily affects visual material, it is reported because of the density of the autobiographical amnesia that was present in the early stages of recovery, the excellent recovery of anterograde memory functioning, and the clarity of the lesion profile on MR imaging.

Case 4.   PM, a right-handed lift engineer (d.o.b. 12 March 1955), suffered a severe head injury in July 1988 as the result of falling down a lift shaft. He suffered a fracture of his anterior fossa, with associated maxillo-facial injuries, and also a collapsed lung. A CT scan showed right frontal and right anterior temporal lobe damage. He was unconscious for 12 days, and "confused" for a further six weeks. In the early stages of recovery, he had some naming difficulties and there were instances of gross confabulation: for example he thought that he had been a soldier who had been blown up in battle and he later thought that a lorry had run over him. His wife thought that his anterograde memory was also impaired in these early stages, but that it returned to near normal around two years after the injury.

He was seen for detailed assessment in 1991. He had some general symptoms, including deafness in the left ear, tension headaches, loss of taste and smell sensation, some double vision when he looked up and scanned horizontally (e.g. when he was viewing balls on a snooker table), and an occasional nasal leak of cerebrospinal fluid. He was also aware of being rather hyperactive, of talking too fast, and having a shorter temper than before his head injury. His wife confirmed these symptoms, and also pointed to occasional word-finding difficulties and a slight disinhibition, especially when talking to others.

Both PM and his wife considered that he did have occasional everyday memory lapses; they also pointed to occasional difficulties in his memory for events that had occurred before his injury and knowledge that had been previously acquired.

Autobiographical Memory Loss.   In the early stages after his head injury, his autobiographical amnesia was severe: for example, for six weeks after regaining consciousness, he did not recognise his wife or his children, thinking that they were his sister's children (he had been married for 13 years). He would sometimes say, "Can somebody get my wife", and when his wife told him that she was his wife he would break down in tears. When he eventually did recognise her as being his wife, he would call her by names other than Babe or Jan—the names he used to call her by before the injury. Several months after the injury, he bought her dark chocolates as a present, seeming to forget completely that she never ate dark chocolates. In the early months of recovery, he also forgot holidays that they had gone on together in the previous few years, and operations that his wife had undergone. She indicated that some of these memories returned 6–9 months after the injury, although it is difficult to say if this was because she repeatedly recounted them to him.

To questioning, PM offered a pre-traumatic amnesia of six hours, and a post-traumatic amnesia of four and a half months. He noted that most of the technical knowledge that he had acquired for his job had been obliterated by his injury, and that he had to relearn this from scratch. For example, when asked a technical question such as what was the "rope stretch" in a lift which he had helped to install, he could not figure this out and had to work it out from scratch over a 30-minute period—usually he would know this "off the top of his head". He indicated that he could recall his early life, in particular his athletic endeavours, and that the clarity of these memories had not changed. He went to New Zealand a few years before the injury, and could recall this, including particular events and the house in which he had lived.

PM was shown family photographs that were taken from an eight-year period prior to his head injury. He was tested on memories that his wife could clearly recall, and which she expected him to recollect:

Photograph from 1980–81: he could recognise his son, but he could not recall having built a wall that was shown in the photograph.
Photograph from Xmas 1982: he could not recognise that this photograph was taken on Xmas day, and he could not recall taking his son to the pond to feed ducks on Xmas day.

Photograph from 1982: he could recognise his son in the photograph, but he could not recall the occasion (being taken to his Christening).

Photograph from 1983: he could not recognise the occasion (a family wedding), but when cued he was able to name some of the people in the photograph.

Photograph from 1986: this was a photograph of the birthday party of his son, prior to their going to New Zealand. He could recognise his son, but he could not recognise the two children from New Zealand who were also in the picture. Neither could he recall meeting their parents, to whom he had spoken at some length.

Photograph from June 1988: this was a photograph of his daughter's birthday party, and it was taken two weeks before the accident. PM did not recall the party from looking at the photograph.

PM was administered the Autobiographical Memory Interview (Kopelman, et al., 1990). His scores on this test were within normal limits—this perhaps reflects the selectivity of his residual autobiographical memory loss, his re-learning of much of the information that he had previously lost, and the fact that a more general structured interview may miss out on specific "islands" of memory loss that may be unique to a particular individual and may only be detectable by using different or more detailed assessment procedures.

Neuropsychological Assessment. On general cognitive tasks, PM did not show any major deficits. On the basis of three verbal subtests (Information, Arithmetic, and Similarities) and three performance subtests (Picture Arrangement, Block Design, and Digit Symbol) from the Wechsler Adult Intelligence Scale–Revised (Wechsler, 1981), he obtained a Verbal IQ of 117, a Performance IQ of 109, and a Full Scale IQ of 115. On the modified Wisconsin Card Sorting Test (Nelson, 1976), he did not show any impairment.

Anterograde memory was assessed using a range of memory tests. His performance on the Revised Wechsler Memory Scale (Wechsler, 1987) was generally above average. He had a Verbal Memory Quotient of 110, a Visual Memory Quotient of 135, a General Memory Quotient of 121, a Delayed Recall Quotient of 111, and an Attention/Concentration Quotient of 110. On a words and a faces recognition memory test (Warrington, 1984), he performed well on the words subtest (48/50), and at a low average level on the faces subtest (41/50).

Brain Imaging. As can be seen in Fig. 3.1, MR scanning showed an extensive lesion in the frontal and temporal lobes of the right hemisphere, with the polar region of each lobe being particularly affected. This was considered to reflect contusional damage suffered as a result of the head

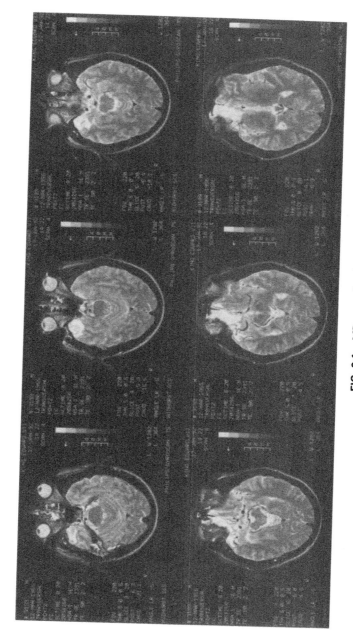

FIG. 3.1. MR scan of patient PM.

injury. There was some enlargement of the right frontal horn, but otherwise no other abnormality was detectable in the rest of the brain. In particular, limbic-diencephalic structures were considered to be intact.

Case 5

BW, a right-handed clerical worker (d.o.b. 27 December 1923), suffered a severe head injury in December 1990 as the result of a road traffic accident in which he was knocked off his cycle by a motor car. An initial skull X-ray showed a right parietal fracture, and a CT scan a few days after the injury showed a right subdural haematoma in the middle fossa, and also haemorrhage within the left temporal and left parietal areas. He also sustained a significant chest injury and fracture of the ribs, but without a pneumothorax. His wife indicated that he was quite confused for around three months after the injury.

When seen in March 1993, he had a pre-traumatic amnesia of around 10 minutes. In the case of post-traumatic amnesia, it was difficult to elicit any period of clear and continuous memory for events subsequent to his injury.

His residual symptoms included memory difficulties, for both pre-injury and post-injury events, some word-finding difficulties, increased irritability, and a greater sensitivity to noise. His wife indicated that he was now prone to major mood swings, with occasional episodes of depression.

Autobiographical Memory Loss.   For practical reasons, a detailed assessment of BW's autobiographical memory was not possible. BW does not recall his children growing up, nor does he recall his children getting married. Six of his eight children have got married, with the first wedding taking place in 1980, 10 years before his head injury. He has no recollection of this or subsequent weddings. He has only patchy memory for the various places in which he worked during his life. He does recall a holiday to Spain that he took with his family in 1973, 17 years before his head injury.

BW's wife also indicated that some trips that he had made in the two years after his injury had been completely forgotten, so it would appear that there is also some post-injury autobiographical memory loss, in spite of the absence of severe impairment on standard anterograde memory tests.

Neuropsychological Assessment.   On general cognitive tasks, BW did not show any major deficits. On the basis of two verbal subtests (Arithmetic and Similarities) and three performance subtests (Picture Arrangement, Block Design, and Digit Symbol) from the Wechsler Adult Intelligence Scale–Revised (Wechsler, 1981), he obtained a Verbal IQ of 97, a Performance IQ of 90, and a Full Scale IQ of 93. On the modified Wisconsin Card Sorting Test (Nelson, 1976), he showed a significant impairment, being unable to attain any categories. His rate of perseverative errors, however, was less than

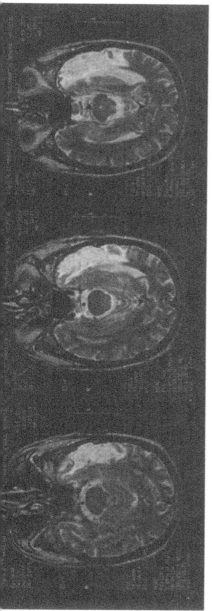

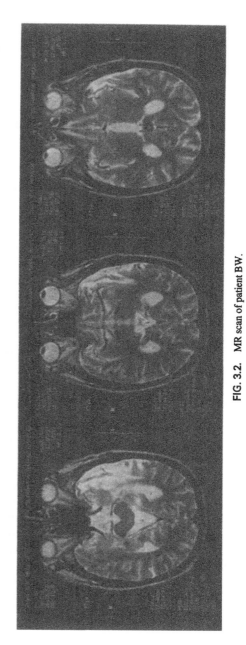

FIG. 3.2.   MR scan of patient BW.

53

50% (36.4%). He had a marked deficit on a picture naming task—the Graded Naming Test (McKenna & Warrington, 1983)—obtaining a score of 3/30. He did not, however, have any major difficulties in general conversational ability during the assessment.

Anterograde memory was assessed using a range of memory tests. His performance on the Revised Wechsler Memory Scale (Wechsler, 1987) showed mild–moderate impairment. He had a Verbal Memory Quotient of 85, a Visual Memory Quotient of 91, a General Memory Quotient of 87, a Delayed Recall Quotient of 92, and an Attention/Concentration Quotient of 110. His limited impairments were evident across most of the subtests, with no particular subtests showing a marked deficit. On a words and a faces recognition memory test (Warrington, 1984), he performed well on the words subtest (44/50 = age-scaled score of 11), and had a mild impairment on the faces subtest (38/50 = age-scaled score of 7).

Brain Imaging.   As can be seen in Fig. 3.2, MR scanning showed major pathology in the left temporal lobe. This was interpreted by a consultant neuroradiologist as showing major loss of brain substance in all three temporal lobe gyri—inferior, middle, and superior temporal lobe gyri—with gliosis in the adjacent white matter. There was also considered to be atrophy of left medial temporal lobe structures such as the hippocampus, but the medial damage was considered to be less severe than the lateral pathology. There was also mild, generalised ventricular dilatation.

Case 6

CH, a 36-year-old right-handed nurse (d.o.b. 8 September 1957), suffered a severe head injury in the USA in July 1988 as the result of falling off a horse. It appears that she had been kicked by the horse in the right fronto-temporal region. A CT scan shortly after the injury showed a left fronto-parietal subdural haematoma that was evacuated. She received ventilation for two weeks. Six weeks later, she was transferred to a hospital in England. Clinical assessment at this time indicated some word-finding difficulties, letter-by-letter reading that impaired her reading of long words, and a right-sided visual field defect. There was also evidence of significant retrograde and anterograde amnesia.

When seen in 1993, she complained of marked memory loss for pre-injury events, but also some anterograde memory difficulties. She was aware of a persistent right visual field defect, and occasional word-finding difficulties. She had a post-traumatic amnesia of around six months. Her pre-traumatic amnesia merged into a more global retrograde amnesia.

Autobiographical Memory Loss.   CH could not recollect events or episodes from most of her pre-injury period, back to her childhood. This

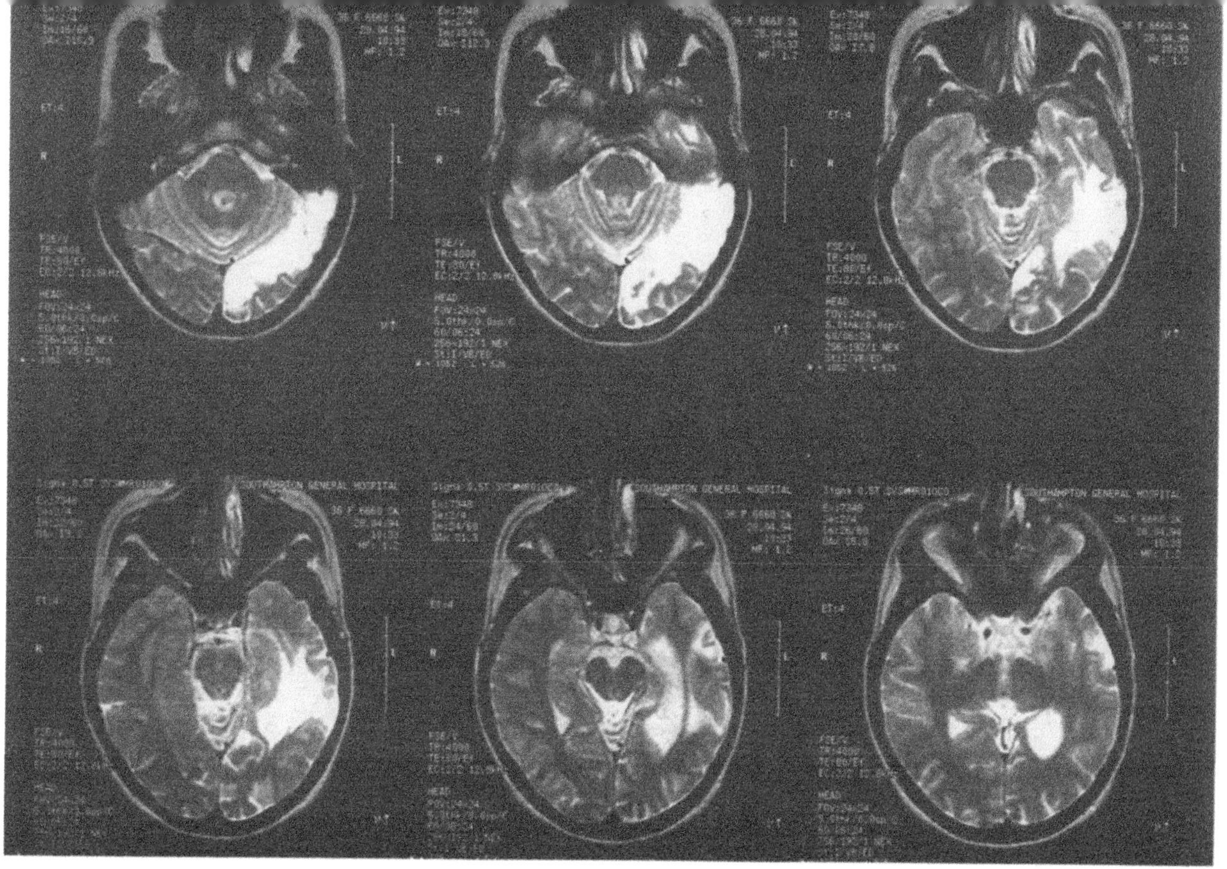

FIG. 3.3. MR scan of patient CH.

autobiographical amnesia included memory loss for the eight years she spent as a nanny in the USA before her head injury, her three years' nursing training from 1976 to 1979, and her time in secondary and primary schools. She had returned to the USA after she recovered from her head injury. She indicated that some faces and places were familiar, but that she could not recollect any specific names or memories associated with these. She also had difficulty in finding her way around familiar places that she knew well before her injury, but after having been there once she could readily relearn the directions. When she was asked to compare her memory for the six years following her head injury with the six years preceding her head injury, CH indicated that the years after her accident were clearer.

On the Autobiographical Memory Interview (Kopelman et al., 1990), she generally performed well on the Personal Semantic items, apart from an abnormal score for Early Adult Life (12.5/21). By contrast, her memory for Autobiographical Incidents was markedly impaired for pre-injury events—thus, her scores for Childhood and Early Adult Life were significantly abnormal (two in both cases).

Neuropsychological Assessment. On the basis of four verbal subtests (Arithmetic, Information, Vocabulary, and Similarities) and four performance subtests (Picture Arrangement, Block Design, Picture Completion, and Digit Symbol) from the Wechsler Adult Intelligence Scale–Revised (Wechsler, 1981), she obtained a Verbal IQ of 85, a Performance IQ of 92, and a Full Scale IQ of 87. Her lowest scores were age-scaled scores of 6 on both the Information and Digit Symbol subtests. On the modified Wisconsin Card Sorting Test (Nelson, 1976), she performed normally. She had a mild deficit on a picture naming task—the Graded Naming Test (McKenna & Warrington, 1983)—obtaining a score of 17/30. On a faces matching task (Benton, Van Allen, Hamsher, & Levin, 1975), she performed normally.

Anterograde memory was assessed using a range of memory tests. Her performance on the Revised Wechsler Memory Scale (Wechsler, 1987) showed mild–moderate impairment. She had a Verbal Memory Quotient of 78, a Visual Memory Quotient of 92, a General Memory Quotient of 81, a Delayed Recall Quotient of 78, and an Attention/Concentration Quotient of 80. On a words and a faces recognition memory test (Warrington, 1984), she also showed mild–moderate impairments (words subtest: 37/50 = age-scaled score of 4; faces subtest: 39/50 = age-scaled score of 7).

Brain Imaging.   As can be seen in Fig. 3.3 MR scanning showed major pathology in the left temporal lobe, stretching back to the left occipital lobe. The temporal lobe damage was considered to include both medial and lateral temporal lobe structures, with posterior portions of temporal lobe gyri being more severely affected than anterior portions. The left thalamus also showed significant abnormality. In addition, there was thought to be limited, milder pathology in the right uncus/entorhinal cortex and right orbitofrontal cortex.

DISCUSSION

I have described six patients, with varying neurological aetiologies, who all presented with autobiographical amnesia as a major feature of their clinical profile. In most instances, there was evidence of temporal lobe pathology. None of the patients had a classical amnesic syndrome. For some patients, in particular those who had suffered a severe head injury, the autobiographical memory loss related primarily to pre-injury events and experiences. However, a few patients, in particular those with temporal lobe epilepsy, complained of memory loss that mainly affected events that had occurred in the months and years previously. Such patients thought that their day-to-day "short-term memory" was relatively intact.

Most of our patients showed some impairment of nonverbal memory, in particular memory for faces. The co-occurrence of autobiographical memory symptoms and nonverbal memory impairment reinforces similar observations from other studies of memory disordered patients. De Renzi, Liotti, and Nichelli (1987) noted that their case, who had mainly left temporal pathology and verbal memory impairment, retained excellent autobiographical memories for past events. Kapur et al. (1992) found that in their patient with bilateral temporal lobe pathology, more marked in the right temporal lobe, and dense retrograde amnesia, the only anterograde impairment of note was a faces memory deficit. In most of the present cases, there was evidence of bilateral temporal lobe involvement, with a small area of gliosis in the right temporal lobe and much more extensive pathology in the left temporal lobe. In the patient LT (Kapur et al., 1992), there was more visible damage to the right anterior temporal lobe, and in the case reported by O'Connor et al. (1992) there was also more extensive damage on the right side. More limited retrograde amnesia, such as that shown by patients with left temporal lobe ablation or epileptogenic lesions (Barr et al., 1990), or after a focal left temporal encephalitic lesion (Yoneda et al., 1992), may be present after unilateral, usually left, temporal lobe damage. More limited, temporally graded retrograde amnesia may also be present in patients with bilateral damage that primarily affects hippocampal structures (Squire, Amaral, & Press, 1990; Squire, Haist, & Shimamura, 1989). Kritchevsky, and Squire (1993) have reported impaired recall performance on a public events retrograde memory test given to three patients whose amnesia was of unknown aetiology, but who appeared to have focal hippocampal damage. Recognition performance was much less impaired in two of the patients. The cerebral pathology in these cases was, however, presumed from reduced volumetric estimates, rather than abnormal MR signals, and it does appear that some degree of ventricular dilatation/generalised atrophy was also present in these three patients. It remains possible that hippocampal damage alone contributes in part to impaired retrograde memory functioning, but this awaits the assessment of patients with well defined, focal hippocampal lesions—single case post-mortem studies have so far indicated only a limited degree of retrograde amnesia after discrete hippocampal pathology (e.g. Victor & Agamanolis, 1990; Zola Morgan, Squire, & Amaral, 1986).

Possible mechanisms underlying autobiographical memory loss after severe head injury have been discussed in earlier papers by the author (Kapur et al., 1992, 1994). The three head injury patients reported in this paper do, however, offer some further insights into this type of amnesia. It is interesting to note that patient BW (Case 5) had a short period of pre-traumatic amnesia that co-existed with a longer-term memory loss for events that he had experienced years before. Thus, this case provides one of the first clinical examples to support a distinction between memory loss for the immediate period preceding the head injury and a more general memory loss for events that may have occurred during a period of months or years prior to the trauma. Williams and Zangwill (1952, p.57) pointed out the possibility of two types of pre-injury amnesia: "(1) A short and usually complete retrograde amnesia; (2) A more diffuse and widely distributed disturbance of memory for pre-traumatic events". The suggestion that a short pre-traumatic amnesia and a more general retrograde amnesia may be dissociable and rely on different neural mechanisms has not been systematically followed up by subsequent research workers, even though it has been acknowledged by other studies of patients with blunt head injury (Benson & Geschwind, 1967) and dates back to the use of the term "retroactive amnesia" by Burnham (1904) and by Talland (1968) to refer to short periods of memory loss for events prior to an insult to the brain.

In cases such as severe head injury, it can reasonably be presumed that diffuse axonal injury will be present to some degree, that there will be *bilateral* pathology, and that temporal lobe structures may be particularly damaged (Kotapka, Graham, Adams, & Gennarelli, 1992). While MR images may only reveal macroscopic, and not microscopic, damage, it is worth noting that two of our head injury cases (Cases 4 and 5, PM and BW) had focal lesions that were unilateral. In one patient, Case 4, these were in the right frontal and temporal lobes, and in the other patient, Case 5, they affected the left temporal region. Case 4 had memory loss that primarily related to loss of visual images of the past, whereas Case 5 appeared to have a more extensive autobiographical amnesia. Thus, it appears possible that different components of autobiographical memory may be affected by right- and left-sided lesions.

Our temporal lobe epilepsy patient (Case 1), who was left with autobiographical amnesia of around 10 years following his epileptic amnesic episode, is very similar to the case reported by Roman-Campos, Poser, and Wood (1980). The duration of retrograde amnesia is similar, and the left temporal lobe EEG focus is also similar in the two cases. Anterograde memory was only minimally impaired in the two patients. The main clinical difference between the two cases is the definitive diagnosis of temporal lobe epilepsy in our patient, and the absence of such a diagnosis in the case reported by Roman-Campos et al. It is possible that longer follow-up in the latter case might have yielded evidence in favour of such a diagnosis. From a consideration of our case, it would appear that an epileptic event may contribute towards a major loss of memory for past events. As epileptic fits are so common in neurological disease, and as our patient's first fit was not a particularly major one, this alone cannot explain the 10-year autobiographical amnesia that ensued. It is quite possible that our patient was experiencing minor epileptic seizures prior to his first fit in 1985, and that these contributed to the episodes of memory loss that he reported in 1984. Thus, it is plausible that a major seizure, combined with a number of earlier minor seizures, which originate from key memory-related structures in the temporal lobe, may play a key role in bringing about a major loss of autobiographical memory that stretches back a number of years.

The autobiographical memory loss shown by our patients with temporal lobe epilepsy contrasts with the minimal or patchy autobiographical memory loss shown by other cases with temporal lobe epileptic lesions who displayed loss of memory for past public events and past knowledge (Ellis, Young & Critchley, 1989; Kapur, Young, Bateman, & Kennedy, 1989). There is no ready explanation for such differences, although they may well be due to the existence of a fractionation within the temporal lobe of particular mechanisms for long-term consolidation of autobiographical events on the one hand and semantic knowledge on the other. The case reported by Ellis et al. (1989) appeared essentially to have an "identification amnesia" that covered people and also other singular items such as buildings and product names. It is also possible that the chronic nature of this condition, compared to the more acute onset of the cases described in this chapter, contributed towards recovery and reorganisation of brain function such that autobiographical memory processes were relatively spared.

Several patients, in particular those with temporal lobe epilepsy, complained of greater memory loss for events that had occurred months or years earlier compared to shorter-term items that had occurred minutes or hours before. This pattern of memory symptoms is rather unusual, but it has been alluded to in some patients with temporal lobe epilepsy. Martin et al. (1991) have remarked on the long-term forgetting shown by temporal lobe epilepsy patients over several days, in comparison to their normal learning of such material over a period of a number of minutes and hours. Empirical study of very long-term retention is obviously difficult to establish in view of the difficulties in obtaining relevant pathological and normal control data over such long time periods.

Three possible mechanisms may underlie our temporal lobe epileptic patients' autobiographical memory loss. First, it is possible that such memory loss reflects the retrograde amnesic effects of clinical epileptic discharges. At one level, this could result from a major seizure bringing about a period of retrograde amnesia, akin to the retrograde amnesic effects of ECT. At another level, it is possible that minor clinical seizures may result in shorter-term retrograde amnesic events (cf. Jus & Jus, 1962), and that over a period of time a large number of such epileptic episodes may have a cumulative effect and lead to a more prolonged period of retrograde amnesia. Thus, in either case, information is considered to have been acquired normally, but is lost owing to the retrograde effects of epileptic events. Second, autobiographical memory loss may be due to impaired long-term consolidation/retrieval processes, ones that govern the consolidation/retrieval of items over months rather than minutes. In this case, the lesion that causes the epilepsy also happens to lead to a defect in the patient's long-term consolidation/retrieval capacity. Third, there may have been impaired learning at the time of the original experience, possibly due to the presence of subclinical discharges that would have affected the consolidation of new information without having any overt effects on behaviour. Thus, information may appear to have been learned normally, and the strength of memory traces that were acquired would have been sufficient for recall after a few minutes/hours, but it is hypothesised that the information had in fact been abnormally acquired, with only partial memory traces being laid down. It remains possible that all three mechanisms may play a part, to a varying extent within particular symptoms and to a variable extent across symptoms, but as yet we have no firm evidence to support the role of one mechanism over any other.

In summary, autobiographical memory loss for longer-term events may be more common as a presenting symptom in neurological disease than has hitherto been acknowledged. It appears to be associated with the presence of temporal lobe pathology, and may be accompanied by nonverbal memory deficits. It may sometimes escape detection in clinical practice unless the clinician specifically asks patients and their carers about long-term memory loss for personally experienced past events.

ACKNOWLEDGEMENTS

I am grateful to the following for their assistance: Mr Roger Johnson, Addenbrooke's Hospital; Mrs Pat Abbott; Dr T.H. Reynolds; Professor Michael Sedgwick; Dr Chris Ellis; Dr Philip Kennedy. I thank the Wellcome Trust for financial support for this research (Grant No. 036191).

REFERENCES

Barr, W.B., Goldberg, E., Wasserstein, J., & Novelly, R.A. (1990). Retrograde amnesia following unilateral temporal lobectomy. *Neuropsychologia*, 28, 243–255.

Benson, D.F., & Geschwind, N. (1967). Shrinking retrograde amnesia. *Journal of Neurology, Neurosurgery and Psychiatry*, 30, 539–544.

Benton, A.L., Van Allen, M.W., Hamsher, K.D., & Levin, H.S. (1975). *Test of facial recognition, Form SL.* Iowa City: Department of Neurology.

Burnham, W.H. (1904). Retroactive amnesia: Illustrative cases and a tentative explanation. *American Journal of Psychology*, 14, 118–132.

Conway, M.A., Rubin, D.C., Spinnler, H., & Wagenaar, W.A. (Eds.), (1992). *Theoretical perspectives on autobiographical memory.* Dordrecht: Kluwer Academic Publishers.

Coughlan, A.K., & Hollows, S. (1985). *The Adult Information Processing Battery.* Leeds: A.K. Coughlan.

Cowles, E. (1900). Epilepsy with retrograde amnesia. *American Journal of Insanity*, 56, 593–614.

Dalla Barba, G., Cipolotti, L., & Denes, G. (1990). Autobiographical memory loss and confabulation in Korsakoff's syndrome: A case report. *Cortex*, 26, 525–534.

Dall'Ora, P., Della Sala, S., & Spinnler, H. (1989). Autobiographical memory. Its impairment in amnesic syndromes. *Cortex*, 25, 197–217.

De Renzi, E., Liotti, M., & Nichelli, P. (1987). Semantic amnesia with preservation of autobiographical memory. A case report. *Cortex*, 23, 575–597.

De Renzi, E., & Lucchelli, P. (1993). Dense retrograde amnesia, intact learning capability and abnormal forgetting rate: A consolidation deficit? *Cortex*, 29, 449–466.

Ellis, A.W., Young, A.W., & Critchley, E. (1989). Loss of memory for people: A case study. *Brain*, 112, 1469–1483.

Goldberg, E., Austin, S.P., Bilder, R.M., Gerstmann, L.J., Hughes, J.E.O., & Mattis, S. (1981). Retrograde amnesia: Possible role of mesencephalic reticular formation in long-term memory. *Science*, 213, 1392–1394.

Hodges, J.R., & McCarthy, R.A. (1993). Autobiographical amnesia resulting from bilateral paramedian thalamic infarction. *Brain*, 116, 921–940.

Jus, A., & Jus, K. (1962). Retrograde amnesia with petit mal. *Archives of General Psychiatry*, 6, 71–75.

Kapur, N. (1993). Focal retrograde amnesia: A critical review. *Cortex*, 29, 217–234.

Kapur, N., Ellison, D., Parkin, A.J., Hunkin, N., Burrows, E., Sampson, S.A., & Morrison, E.A. (1994). Bilateral temporal lobe pathology with sparing of medial temporal lobe structures: Lesion profile and pattern of memory disorder. *Neuropsychologia*, 32, 23–38.

Kapur, N., Ellison, D., Smith, M., McLellan, D.L., & Burrows, E.H. (1992). Focal retrograde amnesia: A neuropsychological and magnetic resonance study. *Brain*, 115, 73–85.

Kapur, N., Young, A., Bateman, D., & Kennedy, P. (1989). Focal retrograde amnesia: A long term clinical and neuropsychological follow-up. *Cortex*, 25, 387–402.

Kopelman, M.D., Wilson, B., & Baddeley, A.D. (1990). The autobiographical memory interview: A new assessment of autobiographical and personal semantic memory in amnesic patients. *Journal of Clinical and Experimental Neuropsychology, 11,* 724–744.

Kotapka, M.J., Graham, D.I., Adams, J.H., & Gennarelli, T.A. (1992). Hippocampal pathology in fatal non-missile human head injury. *Acta Neuropathologica, 83,* 530–534.

Kritchevsky, M., & Squire, L. (1993). Permanent global amnesia with unknown aetiology. *Neurology, 43,* 326–332.

Markowitsch, H.J., Calabrese, P., Liess, J., Haupts, M., Durwen, H.F., & Gelhen, W. (1993). Retrograde amnesia after traumatic injury of the temporo-frontal cortex. *Journal of Neurology, Neurosurgery and Psychiatry, 56,* 988–992.

Martin, R.C., Lorin, D.W., Meador, K.J., Lee, G.P., Thrash, N., & Arena, J.G. (1991). Impaired long-term retention despite normal verbal learning in patients with temporal lobe dysfunction. *Neuropsychology, 5,* 3–12.

McKenna, P. & Warrington, E.K. (1983). *Graded Naming Test.* Windsor, UK: NFER-Nelson.

Nelson, H.E. (1976). A modified card sorting test sensitive to frontal lobe defects. *Cortex, 12,* 313–324.

Nelson, H.E. (1982). *National Adult Reading Test.* Windsor, UK: NFER-Nelson.

O'Connor, M., Butters, N., Miliotis, P., Eslinger, P., & Cermak, L.S. (1992). The dissociation of anterograde and retrograde amnesia in a patient with herpes encephalitis. *Journal of Clinical and Experimental Neuropsychology, 14,* 159–178.

Roman-Campos, G., Poser, C.M., & Wood, F. (1980). Persistent retrograde memory deficit after transient global amnesia. *Cortex, 16,* 500–519.

Squire, L.R., Amaral, D.G., & Press, G.A. (1990). Magnetic resonance imaging of the hippocampal formation and mammillary nuclei distinguish medial temporal lobe and diencephalic amnesia. *Journal of Neuroscience, 10,* 3106–3117.

Squire, L.R., Haist, F., & Shimamura, A.P. (1989). The neurology of memory: Quantitative assessment of retrograde amnesia in two groups of amnesic patients. *Journal of Neuroscience, 9,* 828–839.

Symonds, C. (1962). Concussion and its sequelae. *Lancet, 1,* 1–5.

Talland G.A. (1968). *Disorders of memory and learning.* Harmondsworth, UK: Penguin.

Victor, M., & Agamanolis, D. (1990). Amnesia due to lesions confined to the hippocampus: A clinico-pathologic study. *Journal of Cognitive Neuroscience, 2,* 246–257.

Warrington, E.K. (1984). *Recognition Memory Test.* Windsor, UK: NFER-Nelson.

Wechsler, D. (1981). *Wechsler Adult Intelligence Scale–Revised.* San Antonio, CA: Psychological Corporation.

Wechsler, D. (1987). *Wechsler Memory Scale–Revised.* San Antonio, CA: Psychological Corporation.

Williams, M., & Zangwill, O.L. (1952). Memory defects after head injury. *Journal of Neurology, Neurosurgery and Psychiatry, 15,* 54–58.

Yoneda, Y., Yamadori, A., Mori, E. & Yamashita, H. (1992). Isolated prolonged retrograde amnesia. *European Neurology, 32,* 340–342.

Zola-Morgan, S., Squire, L., & Amaral, D. (1986). Human amnesia and the medial temporal lobe region: Enduring memory impairment following a bilateral lesion limited to field CA1 of the Hippocampus. *The Journal of Neuroscience, 6,* 2950–2967.

4 Focal Retrograde Amnesia: Implications for the Organisation of Memory

Nicola M Hunkin
Royal Hallamshire Hospital, Sheffield, UK

INTRODUCTION

The amnesic syndrome is traditionally defined in terms of a severe anterograde amnesia (AA) accompanied by a variable retrograde amnesia (RA). Thus RA may be minimal, for example in the case of RB (Zola-Morgan, Squire, & Amaral, 1986), or almost total, as in the case of SS (Cermak & O'Connor, 1983). In contrast, a severe AA is considered to be a consistent and necessary feature of the amnesic syndrome and, until recently, it was thought that RA in the absence of AA did not exist. This view, however, has changed as cases of "focal retrograde amnesia" (FRA) have been reported. FRA refers to the presence of a remote memory deficit in the absence of an anterograde deficit, or where the anterograde deficit is considered to be minimal. The occurrence of FRA has important implications for psychological theories of memory. Any such theory must be able to explain how new information may be encoded and retrieved successfully in the context of a failure to recall information from remote memory.

Kapur (1993) has provided a review of FRA cases in the literature. A feature of these cases was the prominence of temporal lobe pathology, which led Kapur to conclude that temporal lobe structures are of importance in mediating FRA. Since publication of Kapur's review, several other cases of FRA have been reported in the literature. Temporal lobe dysfunction has been implicated frequently (Babinsky et al., 1994; Kapur et al., 1994; Markowitsch et al., 1993; Yoneda, Yamadori, Mori, & Yamashita, 1992), but cases of FRA have also been described where there is no apparent evidence of temporal lobe pathology (Brown & Chobor, 1995; De Renzi, Luchelli, Muggia, & Spinnler, 1995).

The existence of FRA, therefore, has implications for two aspects of memory. First, it necessitates consideration of psychological theories of memory in the light of fractionation of amnesic deficits. Second, it allows us to theorise about the neuroanatomy of memory and the relationship between locus of lesion and nature of memory impairment. This chapter describes a case study of FRA resulting from closed head injury. Neuropsychological and neuroradiological data are presented and discussed in the light of these two issues.

CASE HISTORY

DH was born in 1954 and left school at 16 to train as a naval cadet. He became a third officer in the Merchant Navy, but left in 1973 after suffering a closed head injury in a motorcycle accident. Following rehabilitation he had several unskilled jobs before training as a nurse, specialising in mental handicap. After working for a short period as a nurse, he became an instructor on a youth opportunities scheme. In his current job he teaches living skills to young people with learning difficulties, and at weekends he runs a market stall. DH lives with his wife and daughter.

An initial assessment was carried out in 1991. This indicated that DH was an intelligent and fluent speaker with an IQ within the high average range. On tests of verbal memory, his immediate free recall was found to be normal. Delayed recall was in the mild impairment range. There was evidence of more marked impairment on tests of visual memory.

The major deficit presented by DH was his apparent inability to retrieve any memories from the period prior to his accident at age 19. He claimed that he had obtained information from his family about this period, pieced it together, and relearned it. In support of this claim, he gave a convincing account of the difference between genuine memories and those he had relearned as facts. He said it was as if he had read a book about his life but that he did not confuse these facts with real memories any more than one would confuse a story in a book with real life. His wife confirmed that he appeared unable to recall anything from childhood, and reported how he often became distressed by this fact.

NEURORADIOLOGICAL EXAMINATION

Magnetic resonance imaging (MRI) revealed structural lesions in the right parieto-occipital and left occipital lobes. (Details of the MRI protocol together with prints showing extent of the lesions can be seen in Hunkin et al., 1995.)

The left hemisphere lesion involved damage to a discrete area of grey matter on the inferior surface of the occipital lobe, while those in the right hemisphere involved focal atrophy of the cortex and underlying white matter. In addition, there was tissue damage involving the medial surface of the occipital lobes bilaterally. These lesions were associated with some enlargement of the body of the right lateral ventricle and gross enlargement of the posterior horns bilaterally. No focal lesions could be identified in either temporal lobe, and both hippocampi appeared normal. No lesions were visible in the thalamus, but only the right mammillary body could be identified with confidence. Both frontal lobes appeared normal.

NEUROPSYCHOLOGICAL ASSESSMENT

The performance of DH on a range of psychometric tests can be seen in Table 4.1. On the Wechsler Adult Intelligence Test – Revised (WAIS–R; Wechsler, 1981), DH had a pro-rated FSIQ of 111, which was 9 points below that predicted by his performance on the National Adult Reading Test (NART; Nelson, 1991). This depressed IQ score, however, could be accounted for by his poor performance on the digit symbol subtest. Omitting this subtest gave DH an FSIQ score of 117, indicating that he had suffered little intellectual impairment as a result of his injury. On tests of new learning, DH's performance was generally good. On the Wechsler Memory Scale – Revised (WMS–R; Wechsler, 1987) his verbal, visual, and general memory indexes, together with his attention index, were all within one standard deviation (SD) of the population mean, although these indexes were slightly depressed relative to his WAIS–R FSIQ. DH's delayed recall was poorer and was reflected in a delayed memory index of 69. When the WMS–R had been administered, however, it had not been possible to keep to the 30-minute delay recommended. When delayed recall was eventually tested after two hours, DH's performance may have been underestimated. In a follow-up assessment, DH showed similar levels of performance on the immediate tests but showed an improvement on delayed recall, with a delayed memory index that was just over one standard deviation below the population mean. Although there was little difference between DH's WMS–R visual and verbal indexes, on other tests of new learning he tended to perform better on verbal than visual tasks, and showed relative impairment on the faces subtest of the Warrington Recognition Memory Test (WRMT; Warrington, 1984). DH's memory for temporal contextual information was assessed using the list discrimination test (Hunkin, Parkin, & Longmore, 1994). DH's discrimination performance (90%) was similar to the mean (89%) of a group of six age- and IQ-matched control subjects. Frontal lobe functioning was assessed using three tests: Wisconsin Card Sorting Test (WCST; Nelson, 1976), Cognitive Estimation Test (CET; Shallice & Evans, 1978) and Word Fluency (FAS; Benton, Hamsher, Varney, & Spreen, 1983). On all these tests, DH demonstrated normal levels of performance.

EVALUATION OF REMOTE MEMORY DEFICIT

DH's RA was assessed using tests of both public knowledge and personal information. Personal information was tested using the Autobiographical Memory Interview (AMI; Kopelman, 1990). This test provides separate assessments of "personal semantic memory" and memory for "autobiographical incidents". The former comprises knowledge about schools, marriage, children, and career, whereas the latter requires the retrieval of a specific incident (e.g. something that happened at school or at work). DH's performance on this test is shown in Table 4.2. It can be seen that he performed close to normal on all aspects of the test except the childhood component of the autobiographical incidents schedule. On the latter he recalled only one very vague experience involving a plastic coal bucket. It should also be noted that the period sampled by early adult life allowed him to recollect experiences occurring after his accident. In this section DH relied entirely on events from the post-morbid period.

In order to examine DH's autobiographical memory in greater detail he was given the autobiographical cueing procedure devised by Robinson (1976). In this procedure, subjects are given a number of cue words (e.g. river, successful) and are asked to recall a specific personal experience in response to each one. The procedure was administered four times over a period of three years. The results were consistent in that DH was able to produce many specific memories from the post-morbid period, but the only memory he could produce from the pre-morbid period was the coal bucket memory indicated earlier. This pattern of results remained, irrespective of whether DH was allowed to recall from *any* life period or whether he was constrained to recall an event from the pre-morbid period.

In the final administration of the cueing procedure, the specificity, or degree of detail, of DH's recall from the post-morbid period was compared with that of age- and IQ-matched control subjects. The specificity of each recalled episode was rated, on a 5-point scale, by two independent raters. These specificity ratings indicated that DH was impaired relative to controls at producing detailed memories of events. The specificity of his recall for events occurring between the ages of 20 and 26 fell within one standard deviation of the controls, but for the two subsequent six-year periods (age 27–33, 34–40) his specificity was at least two standard deviations below that of the controls.

To assess DH's remote memory for public knowledge, he was given three tests addressing information about famous people and events. These results can be seen in Tables 4.3, 4.4, and 4.5, and in Fig. 4.1. On the Famous Faces Test (Parkin, Montaldi, Leng, & Hunkin, 1990), DH's level of performance was similar to that of age-matched control subjects except for the decade 1966–1975, which covers the period in which he had his accident. On the Famous

TABLE 4.1
DH's Neuropsychological Assessment

NART: 120

WAIS-R	Verbal Tests		Performance Tests	
	Information	12	Picture Completion	12
	Digit Span	14	Picture Arrangement	13
	Arithmetic	12	Block Design	11
	Similarities	12	Digit Symbol	7
	Verbal IQ	118	Performance IQ	102
	Full Scale IQ	111		

WMS-R	Indexes		(follow-up 1994)
	Verbal	96	(97)
	Visual	98	(105)
	General	95	(98)
	Attention	106	(105)
	Delay	69*	(80)

* delay was 2 hours rather than 30 minutes

WRMT				(follow-up 1994)
	Words		47/50	47/50
	Faces		39/50	41/50
	Word–face discrepancy		5–10 percentile	10–25 percentile

RAVLT						
	Trials 1–5	7	9	13	14	13 (max 15)
	After interference	10				
	Delay (30-min)	8				
	Recognition	10 hits, 2 false alarms				

ROCFT		
	Copy	100 percentile
	Immediate	< 10 percentile
	Delay	< 10 percentile

WCST: 6 Categories; 0 Perseverative Errors

CET: 0

FAS: 50

NART: National Adult Reading Test
WAIS–R: Wechsler Adult Intelligence Scale – Revised
WMS–R: Wechsler Memory Scale – Revised
WRMT: Warrington Recognition Memory Test
RAVLT: Rey Auditory-Verbal Learning Test
ROCFT: Rey–Osterrieth Complex Figure Test
WCST: Wisconsin Card Sorting Test
CET: Cognitive Estimation Test
FAS: FAS Word Fluency Test

TABLE 4.2
Performance of DH on the Autobiographical Memory Interview

	Childhood	Young Adult	Recent
Personal Semantic Schedule			
DH	20	20.5	21
Normal Range	16–21	17–21	19–21
Abnormal cut off	≤11	≤14	≤17
Autobiographical Incidents			
DH	1	7	9
Normal Range	6–9	7–9	7–9
Abnormal cut off	≤3	≤3	≤5

Reprinted from *Neuropsychologia, 33*, Hunkin, Parkin, Bradley et al., Focal retrograde amnesia following closed head injury: A case study and theoretical account, 509–523, Copyright (1995), with kind permission from Elsevier Science Ltd, The Boulevard, Langford Lane, Kidlington, OX5 1GB, UK.

Events Test (Parkin & Hunkin, 1991), DH's performance was, again, similar to that of age-matched control subjects, apart from the half-decade corresponding to his accident and the most recent half-decade.

It appears from these data that DH's RA is limited to autobiographical episodic information: performance on tests of personal and public semantic knowledge appears to be relatively well preserved. However, DH claims that he has had to relearn this factual information about himself and about famous people and events. To test this claim, a further test of public knowledge was administered. The aim of this test was to examine DH's knowledge of personalities who were famous for just a short time during the pre-morbid period, and about whom DH would have had little subsequent opportunity to learn. As DH was only 19 years old when he sustained his brain injury, a limited, five-year period was chosen for study in order to maximise the chances that he had previously been familiar with the stimulus names. A list of 95 names was drawn up. Of these, 30 were fictitious names (distractors) and 65 were the names of people who had been famous in the period 1969–1973. Of the 65, roughly half were judged by the experimenter to have been famous only during the specified period (e.g. Iain MacLeod) and half had continued to receive publicity (e.g. Harold Wilson). In order to obtain an objective measure of the extent of fame of a given personality, the list of names was given to six control subjects with a mean age 10 years younger than DH. Subjects were required to indicate whether each name was that of a famous person and, if it was, why that person was famous. This enabled three sets of names to be identified: a set of presumed, decade-specific names (reason for fame given by ≤ 1 control: "HARD" n=32); a set of publicly rehearsed names (reason

TABLE 4.3
Performance of DH and Control Subjects on the Famous Faces Test

		Decade 1956–1965	1966–1975	1976–1985
No context	DH	4	1	3
	Controls	4.2 (1.0)	3.7 (1.5)	4.7 (1.3)
Context	DH	4	3	4
	Controls	4.9 (0.9)	4.5 (1.4)	5.1 (1.0)

Max score = 6. Standard deviations in parentheses.

TABLE 4.4
Performance of DH and Control Subjects on the Public Events Test

	1961–65	1966–70	1971–75	1976–80	1981–85	1986–90
DH	6	6	3	5	7	2
Controls	5.8 (2.1)	5.7 (1.3)	5.9 (2.0)	5.5 (1.9)	6.5 (1.4)	6.1 (1.3)

Max score = 8. Standard deviations in parentheses.

TABLE 4.5
Recognition Performance of DH and Control Subjects on the
Famous Names Test

	d'	FP	TP Easy	TP Medium	TP Hard
DH	0.59	17	16	13	22
Controls	1.60 (0.55)	6.00 (4.73)	15.83 (0.41)	15.17 (0.75)	15.50 (3.83)

TP = true positive responses. FP = false positive responses. Standard deviations in parentheses.

for fame given by ≥ 5 controls: "EASY" n=16; and a set of names with some degree of public rehearsal (reason for fame given by ≥ 4 controls: "MEDIUM" n=17). The set of 95 names was then given to DH and to six age- and IQ-matched controls. Each subject was required to indicate whether each name was that of a famous person and, if it was, to indicate that person's reason for fame.

DH was impaired relative to the controls at identifying the famous names. Table 4.5 shows that his recognition performance was almost two standard deviations below that of the control mean. This poor recognition score was the result of DH making a large number of false positive responses. In contrast, his true positive score was similar to that of controls. Figure 4.1 shows that DH was also poor at identifying reason for fame, and he was impaired relative to controls across all three categories of name. The finding that he was only able to give the reason for fame of 2/32 decade-specific personalities suggests that DH does not have preservation of public semantic information. In contrast, the results are consistent with his claim of having relearned both his personal and public factual knowledge. With increasing opportunity to relearn public information, DH's knowledge improves, although his performance is still impaired relative to controls owing to his mild anterograde deficit.

EVALUATION OF IMAGERY ABILITIES

Recent functional imaging studies have implicated the parietal lobes in memory retrieval (Grasby, Frith, Friston, et al., 1993; Shallice, Fletcher, Frith, et al., 1994). Specifically, activation in the precuneus has been associated with the imagery processes that accompany episodic retrieval. Given that DH has parietal damage, could deficient imagery processes underlie his auto-biographical memory impairment? In an attempt to answer this question, DH was given a number of imagery tests:

1. *Little Men* (Ratcliff, 1979). Subjects were presented with a series (n=32) of 'little men' figures, each on a 4" × 3" card. Each figure held a black disc in one hand. Figures could be presented right way up, upside down, facing out from the card or facing into the card. Subjects were required to indicate in which hand the black disc was. Before starting the test, subjects were given three trials of left-right discrimination. They were presented with a black circle and a white circle side by side, and were required to indicate whether the black circle was on the left or the right. They were also given four practice 'little men' figures to ensure that they understood what was required before commencing the task.

2. *Alphabet Test*. Subjects were given four tasks which required imagery of the letters of the alphabet. In the first task, they were asked to imagine the alphabet in uppercase letters and to tell the examiner all the letters that

contain one or more curved lines (e.g. 'B'). In the second task, subjects were asked to imagine the alphabet in lowercase letters and to tell the examiner all the letters that have stems which go above or below the main body of text (e.g. 'b'). In the third task, they were asked to imagine the alphabet in uppercase letters and to tell the examiner all the letters that have a vertical, straight line on the left hand side (e.g. 'B'). In the fourth task, subjects were required to make a comparison between letters. They heard one letter (e.g. 'A') and were then asked which of two letters ('N' or 'C') was closer in shape to the first letter (i.e. 'N'). There were 20 items in total.

3. *Celebrity Faces* (Hanley, Young, & Pearson, 1991). Subjects were told the name of a famous personality (e.g. Cliff Richard) and then asked which of two personalities (e.g. Mike Read or Noel Edmonds) more closely resembled the first. Prior to administration of this test, the examiner read out all the names which were to be used. Any names not recognised by a subject were excluded from the test.

4. *Clocks* (Grossi, Modafferi, Pelosi, & Trojano, 1989). This test was a modification of the procedure used by Grossi et al. (1989). The examiner read out two clock times (e.g. 20 past 9, 5 to 1). Subjects were required to imagine each of the clock faces and to indicate in which clock face the hands subtended the larger acute angle. There were 20 items in total. Subjects were given practice items before beginning the test, and afterwards they were given a perceptual control test. In the control test, the clock faces (with the same clock times) were presented visually. Subjects were required to make a perceptual judgement indicating in which clock face the hands subtended the larger acute angle.

5. *Verbal description.* Cookie Jar picture (Goodglass & Kaplan, 1983); Scout Camp Picture (Ellis & Young, 1996). As a control task to examine whether DH's verbal description from a picture was as rich and detailed as that of controls, subjects were given two pictures and asked to tell the examiner what was going on in each picture. The narratives were recorded, transcribed and rated by two independent raters on a five-point scale (1 = vague description with no specific detail; 5 = very clear, detailed narrative).

For tasks 1–4, number of errors was recorded and responses were timed.

These tests were designed to tap a number of processes concerned with imagery: ability to perform simple imagery (Alphabet Test); imagery and spatial rotation (Little Men); imagery and comparisons (Clocks, Alphabet Test and Celebrity Faces). DH's performance was compared on each test with a group of age- and NART IQ-matched controls (n=5 for Little Men Test; n=6 for remainder of tests). The results of the imagery tests can be seen in Table 4.6.

The results of the imagery tests indicate that DH has, at the most, a mild impairment in visual imagery. On seven of the above eleven measures, his performance was similar to that of the controls, or within one standard

TABLE 4.6

Peformance of DH and control subjects on tests of
imagery and verbal description

	DH	Controls	
		Mean	SD
Little Men			
% correct	100.00	95.63	3.58
Mean RT	29.84	24.77	4.27
Alphabet Test			
Tasks 1–3: mean no. errors	2.33*	0.61	0.25
Tasks 1–3: mean RT	17.57	19.77	2.47
Task 4: no. errors (max 20)	1.00	0.67	0.82
Celebrity Faces			
% correct	71.43	79.68	10.33
Mean RT per item	4.23*	2.36	0.66
Clocks			
Imagery: no. errors (max 20)	1.00*	0.17	0.41
mean RT per item	3.95	3.65	1.60
Perception: no. errors (max 20)	0.00	0.00	0.00
mean RT per item	1.20	1.67	0.35
Verbal Description			
Rating (1–5)	4.00	3.90	1.40

RT = Reaction time.

* = DH's performance was at least 2 SDs below that of the controls.

deviation of the control mean. Of the three measures on which his performance fell at least two standard deviations below the control mean, two of the measures were error scores. On these two tests, controls seldom made errors. Consequently, a single error in the Clocks Imagery Test meant that DH's performance appeared to be impaired relative to controls. Furthermore, in these timed tasks, there is likely to be a speed-accuracy trade-off. DH appeared to opt for speed on the Alphabet Test with a mean reaction time which was faster than the control mean. His errors on this test were all errors of omission. Finally, his verbal descriptions of the Cookie Jar and Scout Camp pictures were rated as being as detailed as those of the control subjects. In fact both of his descriptions were longer than any of the descriptions given by the control subjects.

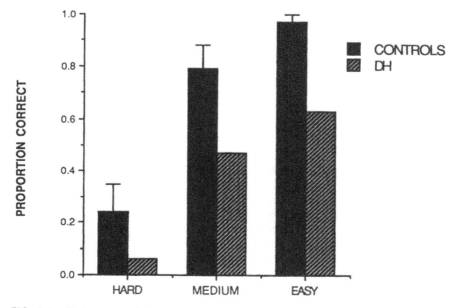

FIG. 4.1. Performance of DH and controls on the Famous Names Test: Ability to identify reason for fame as a function of item difficulty. (Error bars represent one standard deviation.)

Reprinted from *Neuropsychologia*, *33*, Hunkin, Parkin, Bradley et al., Focal retrograde amnesia following closed head injury: A case study and theoretical account, 509–523, Copyright (1995), with kind permission from Elsevier Science Ltd, The Boulevard, Langford Lane, Kidlington, OX5 1GB, UK.

DISCUSSION

DH suffered a closed head injury at the age of 19, but subsequently made a relatively good recovery. When assessed 18 years after his injury, he showed some residual psychomotor slowing and a mild anterograde amnesia. The latter was reflected in some impairment on tests of delayed memory, particularly for non-verbal information. DH's major deficit was an inability to recall any autobiographical incidents from the period prior to his injury. In contrast, he could recall incidents from the period *after* the injury, although the quality of this recall appears to be impoverished relative to that of control subjects. On tests of personal semantic information, DH performed well. Similarly, on two tests of public knowledge (famous faces and famous events), DH performed within normal limits, except for the period around the time of his injury. On a third test of public knowledge, in which DH was asked for information about people who had been famous for a limited time prior to his injury, DH showed a deficit. The results are consistent with DH's claim that he had had to relearn both public and personal information during recovery following his injury.

The results of the imagery tests indicate that, at most, DH may have a mild imagery impairment. His performance on a number of imagery tests was generally within one SD of the control mean, although he tended to perform at the lower end of the control range. It is possible that this mild imagery impairment is related to his diminished vividness in recall of post-morbid events. This diminished vividness does not seem to be accounted for by poverty of verbal descriptions. Although DH's imagery abilities may be related to his quality of post-morbid recall, it is unlikely that such a mild imagery impairment could account for the complete absence of pre-morbid episodic memory.

Before assessing the implications of this case study for neuropsychological and neuroanatomical theories of memory, a diagnosis of psychogenic amnesia had to be considered. This diagnosis seemed unlikely for a number of reasons. First, it is unusual for a functional deficit to persist for as long as 18 years. Second, there were no pre-disposing factors, such as a compensation claim, frequently associated with functional amnesia. Third, there were some signs of organic deficit such as a mild, left-sided hemiplegia and, finally, there was evidence of brain damage on MRI. It was therefore decided that DH's FRA was likely to have an organic basis.

How does this case study of FRA contribute to our understanding of normal memory functioning? First, when considered together with other FRA cases, this study demonstrates the existence of FRA as a distinct clinical disorder. Thus, RA can no longer be considered only as a component of the amnesic syndrome, as severe RA can occur in the context of a minimal anterograde impairment. Second, fractionation of RA itself allows us to examine the dissociation between recall of episodic and semantic information, as researchers have done in investigations of anterograde deficits. Third, consideration of the neuropathology underlying FRA allows us to formulate ideas about the neuroanatomy of memory. Each of these points will be considered in turn.

As a clinical phenomenon, FRA is intriguing because information from the pre-morbid period cannot be recalled, yet new information can be successfully encoded and retrieved. What mechanism(s) can account for this pattern of impairment? The co-occurrence of a severe remote memory deficit with a faster forgetting rate in new learning in their two patients, led De Renzi and Lucchelli (1993) and Maravita, Spadoni, Mazzucchi, and Parma (1995) to suggest that FRA could be accounted for by a consolidation deficit. This view relates to Alvarez and Squire's (1994) proposal that episodic information undergoes long-term consolidation. According to their proposal, storage of episodic information takes place in the neocortex but, initially, retrieval of that information depends upon medial temporal lobe (MTL) structures. As consolidation proceeds, the involvement of medial temporal lobe structures diminishes until the neocortex alone is capable of mediating retrieval. If this consolidation process is impaired, either as a result of MTL or cortical damage, then rate of forgetting will be greater, since information recalled at shorter delays cannot be consolidated and therefore cannot be retrieved at longer delays. It may be argued that DH also has a faster forgetting rate because, on some tests, his anterograde impairment only became apparent on delayed testing. However, a consolidation deficit would predict a temporally-graded retrograde amnesia, since the more remote events would have undergone more consolidation. DH's retrograde amnesia was not temporally graded but covered his entire life before his accident. It is implausible that consolidation necessitates such an extended period, and that childhood memories are dependent upon consolidation processes until at least early adulthood. Furthermore, cases of FRA have been reported in which there is no apparent evidence of an increase in forgetting rate (Babinsky et al., 1994; Kapur, Young, Bateman, & Kennedy, 1989; Yoneda et al., 1992) nor, indeed, evidence of any anterograde deficit (Evans, Breen, Antoun, & Hodges, 1996).

A second explanation may be that FRA represents a storage deficit, such that previously stored information can be erased, leaving the neural substrate functionally intact to store new information. This view, however, is inconsistent with our current understanding of how memory functions. It is thought that memories are stored by changes in synaptic connectivity, embodied in the number and relative strength of synaptic connections. It is implausible that this connectivity can be destroyed, leaving neurones able to acquire new connections. An alternative explanation may be that the connectivity between neurones is only partially degraded. This partial degradation is a pertinent feature of current theories of memory as a distributed system. According to this view, storage of memories occurs over distributed sets of cortical neurones. When learning occurs, connections between sets of neurones become stronger, and subsequent activity in part of a set is more likely to evoke activity in those neurones representing features of the encoded event. If the system is partially degraded then activity in any part of a set of neurones may not reach some threshold level of activity, resulting in failure to recall. However, the system may remain functionally intact and able to relearn old information, and acquire new information, relatively successfully. This would account for the claim (e.g. Brown & Chobor, 1995) that previously known information is re-acquired more quickly than new information. However, this argument fails to account for the relative severity of RA and AA observed in the present case. DH had only a mild AA but he was unable to remember any incidents from the period prior to his injury. It seems implausible that damage that can affect RA so severely causes only a minimal amount of dysfunction in new learning. Furthermore, it is unlikely that the small discrete lesions observed in DH could account for a large storage deficit.

Although it could be argued that DH has additional lesions that were undetected by MRI, it makes little sense to suggest that DH has large areas of dysfunctional neocortex which, nevertheless, allow the storage and retrieval of post-morbid memories.

A further alternative is that DH has a mild storage deficit, which has allowed relearning of pre-morbid public and personal semantic information, but that retrieval of pre-morbid episodic information is denied by an additional "access" or retrieval problem. Thus, it is possible that the substrate of DH's pre-morbid memory has not been destroyed, but that the damage sustained precludes access to memories embodied in this substrate. This can be conceptualised in terms of Damasio's (1989) systems-level model of recall and recognition. According to this model, memory of an event comprises a multi-modal representation of that event. Different aspects of the event are stored as unimodal representations in the sensory cortices in which the event was originally registered, and subsequent recall of the event depends on "time-locked" neural activity within the sensory and motor cortices. Damasio suggests that the coordination of activity in these unimodal cortices depends upon the activation of amodal "convergence zones", some of which are located within the anterior association cortices and limbic system. He suggests that these convergence zones store binding codes, or patterns of synaptic activity, through which information stored within the sensory and motor cortices is accessed. For example, during episodic recall a picture might cue the generation of a visual image, which would activate the binding code generated in the convergence zone at the time the event was experienced. This code, in turn, would activate the other unimodal cortices where other sensory attributes of the event are stored. The binding code would ensure that neural activity generated in the unimodal cortices was time-locked, i.e. that the activity had the same spatial and temporal pattern as that which occurred when the event was experienced. Activity in these unimodal cortices would then be experienced as recall.

This system may breakdown at any one of a number of stages. For example, subjects may not be able to produce a visual image, they may have been unable to generate the binding code in the first place, or there may have been some change in the binding code as a result of damage to brain areas serving as a convergence zone. Damasio's model has been invoked by both O'Connor et al. (1992) and Ogden (1993) to explain the RA observed in their case studies. O'Connor et al. suggested that the FRA observed in their post-encephalitic patient, LD, resulted from damage to the parahippocampal and entorhinal cortices, areas that Damasio (1989) suggested function as amodal convergence zones storing the binding codes. O'Connor et al. suggested that damage to these areas of the brain may modify the binding codes, thereby preventing access to pre-morbidly stored information but, nevertheless, allowing further storage and access of new episodic information. Ogden's (1993) patient, MH, showed a deficit in autobiographical memory, as well as visual and perceptual deficits, following bilateral medial occipital infarction. Ogden suggested that the deficit in autobiographical memory in this patient was a consequence of having to recall an event, stored multi-modally, without the visual aspect of that event. Neither of these explanations can account for the deficit observed in DH, as he has no apparent evidence of parahippocampal or entorhinal damage, there is no evidence of a substantial imagery impairment, and he is able to recall episodes from the post-morbid period (although the degree of detail available in these memories is inferior to that of controls). However, DH's pattern of deficits may be explained if his brain injury resulted in a change in the nature of the code underlying the visual representation, or in the transmission of either this visual code or the binding code. An analogy may be drawn with infantile amnesia where it has been suggested (Perner, 1992) that memories during the first years of life are encoded in such a way that access is denied to the retrieval mechanisms operational in adult life. It is suggested that DH's lesions disrupt transmission of information either to the convergence zones from visual/imagery activity in the posterior cortex, or to the posterior cortex from the convergence zones. Disruption of either of these processes would result in the failure to generate synchronised activity in the unimodal cortices that was similar to that present at the time of the original event. Recall would, therefore, be denied. However, if disruption of these processes was not total, then residual activity in this pathway would enable the visual cortex and convergence zones to communicate sufficiently to set up new, albeit less efficient, binding codes and allow storage and retrieval of new memories.

This retrieval explanation of DH's RA is consistent with the view put forward by Kapur, Scholey, Moore, et al. (1996). Using a similar framework to that of Damasio (1989), Kapur and colleagues suggest that memory retrieval involves the reactivation of representations located in many different cortical sites. They propose that activation memory mechanisms act upon stored representations, of which there are two types: those that store perceptual features (feature codes) and those that store contextual markers (index codes). They suggest that feature codes are located in association cortex, in temporal, parietal and occipital areas, whereas index codes are stored in anterior and inferior temporal cortex. Damage to both types of code, or the transmission of information between brain regions representing these codes, can lead to a deficit in autobiographical memory. Thus, FRA may result from damage to a combination of critical anterior and posterior cortical sites or the connections between them. This would account for the varied pathology reported in different cases of FRA.

The retrieval explanation of DH's RA makes different predictions from a storage deficit explanation. A storage deficit explanation of RA would predict that stimuli of different modalities would be equally poor at evoking pre-morbid memories in DH. However, according to Damasio's model outlined earlier, auditory, olfactory, and tactile stimuli would be more likely to evoke a pre-morbid memory than a visual stimulus, although the memory is still likely to be impoverished without a visual component. Of note is Ogden's (1993, p.588) comment that in her patient, MH, events that are recalled involve "smell, taste and strong emotional reactions". Similarly, DH reported that his one "memory" from the time before his injury, the vague recall of the blue plastic coal bucket, was associated with the grating sound of a coal shovel. Furthermore, DH reported that in checking the veracity of autobiographical recall (from the post-morbid period), he judges whether the events have smells or sounds associated with them.

So far we have considered explanations for the phenomenon of FRA as observed in DH. What does the study of DH tell us about the fractionation of RA? On initial testing, DH seemed to show a clear distinction between impaired performance on tests of autobiographical episodic information (AMI: Autobiographical Incidents, Robinson technique), and performance on tests of personal and public knowledge, which was relatively intact (AMI: Personal Semantic Schedule, Famous Faces, Famous Events). This is consistent with other studies of FRA that have reported a dissociation between these two aspects of memory. Kapur et al. (1989) described a patient who showed poor performance on tests of public knowledge but who had relative preservation of autobiographical memory. Other studies (Babinsky et al., 1994; Markowitsch et al., 1993; O'Connor et al., 1992; Stracciari et al., 1994) have shown the converse, describing patients with severe autobiographical memory deficits who show relative preservation of personal and/or public semantic information. Whether the latter cases simply reflect the relearning of information that had been known prior to the illness/injury should be considered. DH's performance on the Famous Names Test is consistent with this possibility because he showed impairment in identifying people and their occupations when those people's exposure in the media had been limited to the pre-morbid period. Certainly, in the 18 years since his accident, DH would have had opportunity to learn about people and events featured in the first two tests. In the cases reported by O'Connor et al. (1992) and Markowitsch et al. (1993) it appears that testing of remote memory took place eight and four years post-illness/injury, respectively, thus allowing opportunity for relearning of public semantic information. However, this explanation cannot account for the dissociation observed in Babinsky et al.'s (1994) patient who was tested 15 days after onset of neurological symptoms. Thus, dissociation between semantic and episodic remote memory should be considered, although DH lends no direct support to this issue.

Finally, what can the neuropathology underlying DH's FRA tell us about the organisation of normal memory? Previous reports of FRA have highlighted the importance of the temporal lobes in remote memory functioning. In particular, remote memory deficits have been associated with anterior temporal lobe damage (Kapur et al., 1992, 1994; Markowitsch et al., 1993) although posterior temporal lobe dysfunction has also been implicated (De Renzi & Lucchelli, 1993; Yoneda et al., 1992). In the present case, MRI showed no evidence of temporal lobe pathology but indicated damage to the right parieto-occipital lobe and occipital lobes bilaterally. Similarly, Brown and Chobor (1995) found no temporal lobe damage in their patient, MM, who had lesions involving the right frontal and left occipital lobes. Although the use of the term FRA to describe MM's pattern of memory impairment is not strictly justified, her remote memory was considered to be disproportionate to her anterograde impairment. This discrepant neuropathology may be accommodated within Damasio's framework if the critical lesions disrupt different stages of the retrieval process. Temporal lobe lesions, for example, may directly damage the convergence zones, thereby preventing reinstatement of the binding code essential for recollection. Parieto-occipital lesions, on the other hand, may disrupt input to, or output from, the convergence zones. This would effectively alter the correspondence between the convergence zones and the unimodal cortices. DH's particular pattern of memory impairment, ability to recall post-morbid events in the complete absence of pre-morbid recall, may then be explained by a renegotiation between convergence zones and unimodal cortices. Thus, brain trauma may have damaged the interaction between convergence zones and unimodal cortices, but residual activity has allowed new binding codes to be established, thereby enabling new interactions to be made.

CONCLUSION

The study of DH has provided us with valuable information about FRA. DH demonstrated a severe deficit in the ability to recall personal events from the period prior to his injury. In contrast, he showed only a mild anterograde impairment, evident largely on delayed testing, and could recall incidents from the *post*-morbid period. His performance on tests of remote memory for personal and public semantic information appeared to be preserved, but it is concluded that DH's performance on these tests reflects relearning of this information in the time since his injury. This study has enabled us to challenge the view that temporal lobe damage is critical to FRA and allowed us to speculate on the nature of the dysfunction caused by DH's occipital and parieto-occipital lesions. It is concluded that a storage deficit explanation is insufficient to account for DH's remote memory deficit. An alternative retrieval explanation is proposed, which is expressed in terms of Damasio's (1989) multiregional retroactivation framework.

ACKNOWLEDGEMENTS

The study of DH was carried out in collaboration with A.J. Parkin, V.A. Bradley, E.H. Burrows, F.K. Aldrich, A. Jansari, C. Burdon-Cooper, and E.J. Squires, and was supported by the Wellcome Trust (Grant number 037666). I am grateful to DH for giving up time to take part in this study. Thanks also to Claerwen Snell and Cath Brown for help with collection of control data and to Jim Stone for comments on the text.

REFERENCES

Alvarez, P., & Squire, L.R (1996). Memory consolidation and the medial temporal lobe: A simple network model. *Proceedings of the National Academy of Sciences, 91*, 7041–7045.

Babinsky, R., Maier, B., Calabrese, P., Markowitsch, H.J., & Gehlen, W. (1994). Atraumatic temporal lobe pathology and autobiographical memory. *European Neurology, 34*, 290–291.

Benton, A.L., Hamsher, K., Varney, N., & Spreen, O. (1983). *Contributions to neuropsychological assessment.* New York: Oxford University Press.

Brown, J.W., & Chobor, K.L. (1995). Severe retrograde amnesia. *Aphasiology, 9*, 163–170.

Cermak, L.S., & O'Connor, M. (1983). The anterograde and retrograde retrieval ability of a patient with amnesia due to encephalitis. *Neuropsychologia, 21*, 213–234.

Damasio, A.R. (1989). Time-locked multiregional retroactivation: A systems-level proposal for the neural substrates of recall and recognition. *Cognition, 33*, 25–62.

De Renzi, E., & Lucchelli, F. (1993). Dense RA, intact learning capability and abnormal forgetting rate: A consolidation deficit? *Cortex, 29*, 449–466.

De Renzi, E., Lucchelli, F., Muggia, S., & Spinnler, H. (1995). Persistent retrograde amnesia following a minor trauma. *Cortex, 31*, 531–542.

Ellis, A.W., & Young, A.W. (1996). *Human cognitive neuropsychology: A textbook with readings.* Hove, UK: Psychology Press.

Evans, J.J., Breen, E.K., Antoun, N., & Hodges, J.R. (1996). Focal retrograde amnesia for autobiographical events following cerebral vasculitis: A connectionist account. *Neurocase, 2*, 1–11.

Goodglass, H., & Kaplan, E. (1983). *The Boston Diagnostic Aphasia Examination.* Philadelphia: Lea and Febiger.

Grasby, P.M., Frith, C.D., Friston, K.J., Bench, C., Frackowiak, R.S.J., & Dolan, R.J. (1993). Functional mapping of brain areas implicated in auditory-verbal memory function. *Brain, 116*, 1–20.

Grossi, D., Modafferi, A., Pelosi, L., & Trojano, L. (1989). On the different roles of the cerebral hemispheres in mental imagery: The "o'Clock Test" in two clinical cases. *Brain and Cognition, 10*, 18–27.

Hanley, J.R., Young, A.W., & Pearson, N. (1991). Impairment of the visuo-spatial sketch pad. *Quarterly Journal of Experimental Psychology, 43A*, 101–125.

Hunkin, N.M., Parkin, A.J., Bradley, V.A., Burrows, E.H., Aldrich, F.K., Jansari, A., & Burdon-Cooper, C. (1995). Focal retrograde amnesia following closed head injury: A case study and theoretical account. *Neuropsychologia, 33*, 509–523.

Hunkin, N.M., Parkin, A.J., & Longmore, B.E. (1994). Aetiological variation in the amnesic syndrome: Comparisons using the list discrimination task. *Neuropsychologia, 32*, 819–825.

Kapur, N. (1993). Focal retrograde amnesia in neurological disease: A critical review. *Cortex, 29*, 217–234.

Kapur, N., Ellison, D., Parkin, A.J., Hunkin, N.M., Burrows, E.H., Sampson, S.A., & Morrison, E.A. (1994). Bilateral temporal lobe pathology with sparing of medial temporal lobe structures: Lesion profile and pattern of memory disorder. *Neuropsychologia, 32,* 23–38.

Kapur, N., Ellison, D., Smith, M., McLellan, L., & Burrows E.H. (1992). Focal retrograde amnesia following bilateral temporal lobe pathology: A neuropsychological and magnetic resonance study. *Brain, 115,* 73–85

Kapur, N., Scholey, K., Moore, E., Barker, S., Brice, J., Thompson, S., Shiel, A., Cam, R., Abbott, P., & Fleming, J. (1996). Long-term retention deficits in two cases of disproportionate retrograde amnesia. *Journal of Cognitive Neuroscience, 8,* 416–434.

Kapur, N., Young, A., Bateman, D., & Kennedy, P. (1989). Focal retrograde amnesia: A long term clinical and neuropsychological follow-up. *Cortex, 25,* 387–402.

Kopelman, M.D. (1990). *Autobiographical Memory Interview.* Reading, UK: Thames Valley Test Company.

Maravita, A., Spadoni, M., Mazzucchi, A., & Parma, M. (1995). A new case of retrograde amnesia with abnormal forgetting rate. *Cortex, 31,* 653–667.

Markowitsch, H.J., Calabrese, P., Liess, J., Haupts, M., Durwen, H.F., & Gehlen, W. (1993). Retrograde amnesia after traumatic injury of the fronto-temporal cortex. *Journal of Neurology, Neurosurgery and Psychiatry, 56,* 988–992.

Nelson, H.E. (1976). A modified card sorting test sensitive to frontal lobe defects. *Cortex, 12,* 313–324.

Nelson, H.E. (1991). *National Adult Reading Test* (2nd Edn.) Windsor, UK: NFER Nelson.

O'Connor, M., Butters, N., Miliotis, P., Eslinger, P., & Cermak, L.S. (1992). The dissociation of anterograde and retrograde amnesia in a patient with Herpes encephalitis. *Journal of Clinical and Experimental Neuropsychology, 14,* 159–178.

Ogden, J.A. (1993). Visual object agnosia, prosopagnosia, achromatopsia, loss of visual imagery and autobiographical amnesia following recovery from cortical blindness: Case M.H. *Neuropsychologia, 31,* 571–589.

Parkin, A.J., & Hunkin, N.M. (1991). Memory loss following radiotherapy for nasal pharyngeal carcinoma—An unusual presentation of amnesia. *British Journal of Clinical Psychology, 30,* 349–357.

Parkin, A.J., Montaldi, D., Leng, N.R.C., & Hunkin, N.M. (1990). Contextual cueing effects in the remote memory of alcoholic Korsakoff patients and normal subjects. *Quarterly Journal of Experimental Psychology, 42A,* 585–596.

Perner, J. (1992). Grasping the concept of representation: Its impact on 4-year-olds' theory of mind and beyond. *Human Development, 35,* 146–155.

Ratcliff, G. (1979). Spatial thought, mental rotation and the right cerebral hemisphere. *Neuropsychologia, 17,* 49–54.

Robinson, J.A. (1976). Sampling autobiographical memory. *Cognitive Psychology, 8,* 578–595.

Shallice, T., & Evans, M.E. (1978). The involvement of the frontal lobes in cognitive estimation. *Cortex, 14,* 294–303.

Shallice, T., Fletcher, P., Frith, C.D., Grasby, P., Frackowiak, R.S.J., & Dolan, R.J. (1994). Brain regions associated with acquisition and retrieval of verbal episodic memory. *Nature, 368,* 633–635.

Stracciari, A., Ghidoni, E., Guarino, M., Poletti, M., & Pazzaglia, P. (1994). Post-traumatic retrograde amnesia with selective impairment of autobiographical memory. *Cortex, 30,* 459–468.

Warrington, E.K. (1984). *Recognition Memory Test.* London: NFER Nelson.

Wechsler, D. (1981). *Wechsler Adult Intelligence Scale – Revised.* New York: Psychological Corporation.

Wechsler, D. (1987). *Wechsler Memory Scale – Revised*. New York: Psychological Corporation.

Yoneda, Y., Yamadori, A., Mori, E., & Yamashita, H. (1992). Isolated prolonged retrograde amnesia. *European Neurology, 32*, 340–342.

Zola-Morgan, S., Squire, L.R., & Amaral, D.G. (1986). Human amnesia and the medial temporal region: Enduring memory impairment following a bilateral lesion limited to field CA1 of the hippocampus. *Journal of Neuroscience, 6*, 2950–2967.

5 Lost for Words: A Case of Primary Progressive Aphasia?

Kim S. Graham
Addenbrooke's Hospital, Cambridge, UK
MRC Applied Psychology Unit, Cambridge, UK

James T. Becker
University of Pittsburgh Medical Center, USA

Karalyn Patterson
MRC Applied Psychology Unit, Cambridge, UK

John R. Hodges
Addenbrooke's Hospital, Cambridge, UK
MRC Applied Psychology Unit, Cambridge, UK

INTRODUCTION

Patients with neurodegenerative disease may present with relatively focal symptoms such as a loss of spoken language ability (aphasia). In 1892, Arnold Pick reported a 71-year-old man with a profound progressive aphasia evolving into a more generalised loss of mental abilities (dementia), who at post-mortem showed pronounced shrinkage of the left temporal lobe. By 1914, Mingazzini, an Italian neurologist, summarised the findings of 16 similar cases from the European literature. Following this initial flurry of reports there was a gradual waning of interest until the early 1980s when Mesulam (1982) again drew attention to the phenomenon of what he termed slowly progressive aphasia without generalised dementia. Since then, almost 100 other patients have been described who conform to the diagnostic criteria for "primary progressive aphasia" as proposed by Mesulam and Weintraub (1992): a progressive deterioration of language with preservation of the activities of daily living for at least two years, and evidence of relatively normal non-verbal abilities on neuropsychological testing (Caselli et al., 1992; Hodges, Patterson, Oxbury, & Funnell, 1992a; Hodges, Patterson, & Tyler, 1994; Mesulam & Weintraub, 1992; Parkin, 1993; Poeck & Luzzatti, 1988; Scheltens, Ravid, & Kamphurst, 1994; Snowden, Goulding, & Neary, 1989; Snowden et al., 1992; Tyrrell, Warrington, Frackowiak, & Rossor, 1990).

Although essentially all patients with primary progressive aphasia share deficits in naming objects and in producing words at will in conversation, the literature suggests that there are in fact two major sub-types with radically different underlying cognitive deficits: progressive fluent aphasia (also coined semantic dementia, Hodges et al., 1992a; Snowden et al., 1989) and progressive nonfluent aphasia (Hodges & Patterson, 1996). In patients with the fluent form, the language difficulties can most often be attributed to a selective impairment of semantic memory. The term semantic memory refers to our knowledge about objects and the meanings of words, concepts, and facts. This knowledge is crucial to our understanding of the world around us and is involved in many different cognitive processes. Breakdown of semantic memory results in a loss of word and object meaning, impoverished general knowledge, reading and writing difficulties, and profound anomia for previously familiar words and names. Loss of semantic information does not, at least initially, affect phonological, grammatical (syntactic), or prosodic (melodic and intonational) aspects of the patients' speech. A typical case of progressive fluent aphasia with severe semantic deterioration (JL: Hodges et al., 1992a; Hodges, Graham, & Patterson, 1995) will be described later.

The language disturbance in progressive nonfluent aphasia is strikingly different: patients show no significant loss of semantic knowledge or impairment on tests of single-word comprehension. Instead they have a progressive breakdown in the phonological and syntactic domains of language, which causes distorted spontaneous speech, frequent phonological paraphasias (e.g. producing "lawnlower" for *lawnmower*), numerous word-finding pauses, and difficulty repeating words and phrases (Croot, Patterson, & Hodges, in press; Hodges & Patterson, 1996). In both forms of progressive aphasia, visuo-spatial, perceptual, and non-verbal problem-solving abilities remain intact and patients have good day-to-day (episodic) memory (see Hodges & Patterson, 1996; Karbe, Kertesz, & Polk, 1993; Mesulam & Weintraub, 1992).

In addition to these two major, frequently described, patterns of primary progressive aphasia, there have been occasional reports of progressive language deterioration that do not fit either sub-type. For example, a patient (FM) originally described by Hodges et al. (1992a) as a case of fluent progressive aphasia with mild semantic loss showed a subsequent pattern of deterioration that was highly atypical of this sub-type: her speech remained fluent and her anomia became even more profound, but, in contrast to patients like JL mentioned earlier, her mild semantic abnormality remained largely static and therefore seemed an unlikely source of her deteriorating language abilities. Graham, Patterson, and Hodges (1995) attributed FM's "progressive pure anomia" to a reduction in communication between semantic and phonological representations.

In this chapter, we describe a recently studied patient (GC) who presented with a difficulty "remembering" the names of people, local places, and objects. He also had problems understanding the meaning of words that had been previously familiar to him. We discuss the nature of his language disorder with respect to the two patients described in this introduction, JL and FM, both of whom showed similar problems in word-finding at presentation. The question addressed is whether GC's pattern is most adequately considered as an example of semantic dementia or of progressive pure anomia; our attempts to elucidate the nature of his naming problems illustrate, we hope, an appropriate use of the single-case methodology in cognitive neuropsychology.

SEMANTIC DEMENTIA: JL

JL was a 61-year-old successful self-employed businessman. For three years prior to his initial neurological consultation in 1991, he had increasing difficulty remembering the names of friends, colleagues, and local places (including those he frequently visited during a working week). For example, his family reported noticing that he had difficulty producing the names of his employees when compiling their weekly pay packets. This anomia was quite severe on formal picture naming assessments: on a picture naming test consisting of 48 line drawings of familiar animals and manmade items (see Hodges, Salmon, & Butters, 1992b), JL named 17 (35%) when first tested; a year later, he could name only five (10%) of the items; appropriately matched controls obtained an average score of 43.6 (± 2.3) in a speeded (computerised) version of the naming test.

A detailed analysis of JL's picture naming over a period of about 1.5 years, based on all 260 pictures from the Snodgrass and Vanderwart (1980) corpus of line drawings, revealed that JL's failure to name an item on one occasion virtually always meant that he would be unable to name it when next tested (Hodges et al., 1995). In addition, there was a consistent trend in the type of errors produced: for instance, in response to pictures of animals he initially produced a range of category exemplar errors ("pig" for kangaroo; "elephant" for rhinoceros), but gradually his responses became stereotyped and consisted of only highly prototypical category members ("cat", "dog", "horse"), and eventually even these were replaced by the superordinate response "animal". He also showed a significant inter-test consistency between his ability to name items and to describe them from their names on five separate sessions. This pattern of performance on picture naming (and also comprehension) tests suggests that JL was gradually losing specific features from the conceptual knowledge base that allows normal subjects to identify and differentiate between semantically similar animals and objects.

JL's performance on other tests of semantic memory showed a parallel decline over a two-year period. For example, on a word–picture matching test where the subject must pick out the correct picture from among eight semantically similar exemplars (e.g. zebra with seven other four-legged large animals) in response to the spoken name, JL's performance dropped rapidly (31/48 to 10/48 vs controls 47.4 ± 1.1). Another test of semantic memory is the Pyramids and Palmtrees Test (Howard & Patterson, 1992), which can be given in various picture- or word-based formats: in the three-picture version, the subject points to one of two pictures that goes best with a target (for example, target = *windmill*, related item = *tulip*, foil = *daffodil*). While controls score virtually perfectly, JL, when first tested in April 1991, chose only 36/52 (69%) of the correct alternatives. By September 1992, this had deteriorated to chance performance (50% correct).

The fact that JL's loss of semantic knowledge extended to other domains of non-verbally based semantic memory was confirmed using a range of tasks. For example, JL had profound difficulty when colouring-in black-and-white line drawings of common items, such as tomato (coloured blue) and crocodile (yellow). He correctly coloured 20% of the 40 items, while control subjects select appropriate colours for 75–95% of these items. By contrast, he showed no decline on tests tapping basic perceptual and visuo-spatial abilities. For example, he scored 95% in copying the complex Rey Figure (Osterrieth, 1944) in April 1991 and 89% in October 1992. Reasonably stable performance was also seen on tests of non-verbal problem solving and of short-term memory.

PROGRESSIVE PURE ANOMIA: FM

FM was a 55-year old woman with a 12-month history of difficulty with word production, especially for people's names and everyday objects. This had initially become apparent at her place of work, an old people's home, where she started to experience problems telling residents what was for lunch, dinner etc. and in relaying reports about residents to other staff members. She was originally thought to be at an early stage of the syndrome of semantic dementia (Hodges et al., 1992a); but in retrospect it became clear that, on any test of semantic memory that did not rely on spoken word production (e.g. word–picture and picture–picture matching etc.), her degree of impairment was, at most, mild. Her deficits were confined to the language domain; she remained capable of running the house (shopping, cooking etc.), looked after her sick husband and was active in church affairs. Her day-to-day memory was excellent: she easily remembered appointments and social engagements, and could recall events that had happened in the recent past. For example, during the time FM was tested, she never showed any difficulty remembering specific events from her holidays and visits to relatives etc. Her performance on tests of perceptual, visuo-spatial, and non-verbal problem solving was also excellent.

During the first three years of follow-up, FM showed a progressive deterioration on all tests that required spoken word production: picture naming, naming in response to a verbal description (e.g. "what do we call the large grey animal with a trunk?"), and category fluency (where the subject produces as many items as possible in one minute from given categories such as animals, household items etc.). This decline, however, was not accompanied by any further loss of semantic knowledge: her performance on tests of single-word comprehension remained stable. For example, while JL deteriorated significantly on the spoken word–picture matching test over a two-year period (31/48 to 10/48), FM's score did not change over the first three years she was tested (see Fig. 5.1). She showed similarly stable

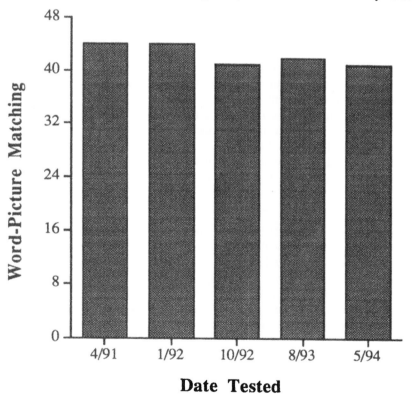

FIG. 5.1.   FM's performance on the Hodges et al. (1992b) word–picture matching test (n=48) over time (April 1991–May 1994).

performances on other tasks that assess semantic memory, such as a picture sorting test, in which the subject is asked to sort pictures of animals and objects into groups according to a set of criteria that vary in difficulty (e.g. manmade/living; land animals/birds/water creatures; fierce/not fierce etc.). Most recently, she has shown some deterioration in her syntactic abilities and on some more difficult tests requiring her to combine the meanings of words (Tyler, Moss, Patterson, & Hodges, 1997).

These observations suggested that the functional locus of FM's naming difficulty was not at the level of the semantic system, but rather a reduced ability to activate appropriate phonological word forms in the lexicon for speech production. A disruption of representations within the phonological lexicon itself seemed unlikely, as FM never made phonological speech errors and had no problems in immediate repetition of even multisyllabic words. To investigate the hypothesis that FM's anomia resulted from pathologically reduced activation of phonology by semantics, we applied the gating methodology (see Tyler, 1992, Chapter 5) in which subjects are asked to produce a word upon hearing successively larger fragments. For example, for the target word *centipede*, the subject hears the first 100ms of the word (roughly "se"), then the first 150ms ("sen"), then the first 200ms ("sent"), and so on, until the subject is able to identify the word. "Centipede" is typically recognised once "sentip_" is detected, as there are no other words in English that have this sensory sequence. The full results are reported elsewhere (Graham et al., 1995) but, in brief, these studies supported the hypothesis that FM's anomia was attributable to a deficit in communication between semantic memory and the phonological system. For instance, FM showed only minimal benefit when the normal phonetic sequence in the gating task was accompanied by simultaneous presentation of a picture of the target word.

CASE STUDY: GC

GC was a 57-year-old, right-handed former executive in a large manufacturing company, who presented with word-finding difficulties. His wife reported that up to four years prior to his presentation he had also shown some minor behavioural changes: he was less likely to engage in social activities and had some problems organising and documenting work.

GC's spontaneous speech, although marked by word-finding pauses, was fluent with normal syntax and phonology. His word-finding problem was evident for previously familiar common nouns and verbs, as well as the names of people and places. For example, he could name only 118 (45%) of the 260 pictures in the Snodgrass and Vanderwart (1980) corpus. Like the two previous cases (see Graham, Hodges, & Patterson, 1994 for more detail), the majority of GC's errors on tests of picture naming were semantic or visual/semantic: he produced superordinates ("animal" for *leopard*), semantic substitutions ("boot" for *shoe*) and circumlocutions ("to put on my feet" for *sock*; "use it over there and put bread in it" for *toaster*). In addition, and again like the two previous cases, GC's picture naming was influenced by word frequency: he was more successful on pictures with names high in frequency than on pictures with low-frequency names (Graham et al., 1994).

GC's performance on other tests thought to assess semantic knowledge showed a variable degree of impairment, perhaps related to modality of stimulus presentation/response (an issue discussed at greater length later). On a category fluency test, where he was given one minute to produce as many exemplars as possible from various specified categories (i.e. animals, birds, vehicles, musical instruments etc.), GC produced only 6 examples for the animal category, compared to controls who produce on average 18 (± 3.8). His performance on other categories was equally poor. His semantic deficit was also evident on various versions of a 106-item word–picture matching test, in which the subject is asked to select the correct item (e.g. brick) from amongst four foils: one close semantic (rock), one distant semantic (wall), one phonological (chick) and one visual (luggage trunk). GC's performance on this test, although not profoundly impaired, was clearly below normal and below his pre-morbid ability (only 80–85% of items were correctly matched whereas controls perform almost perfectly). He was also impaired on tests of synonym judgement in which the subject has to decide which two words out of a set of three are closest in meaning: for example, on the written version from the Psycholinguistic Assessment of Language Processing in Aphasia (PALPA, Kay, Lesser, & Coltheart, 1992) he scored well below the control range (68%). By contrast, on a semantic test involving only pictures (the Pyramids and Palmtrees Test, three-picture version), he scored 47 (90%), which is not quite normal (control subjects select 98–99% of the items correctly) but represents a very mild impairment.

His day-to-day memory and autobiographical memory seemed relatively unaffected by his illness, and both visuo-spatial skills and recall of simple verbal material were normal. GC showed no disorientation in time and place and no impairment on digit span tests (6 forwards).

A coronally orientated MRI scan (taken on 6/94) showed striking, selective atrophy to the left temporal neocortex, involving the inferior and middle temporal gyri with relative preservation of the hippocampal formation (see Fig. 5.2).

A COMPARISON OF THE NEUROPSYCHOLOGICAL PROFILES OF THE THREE PATIENTS

Table 5.1 illustrates a sample of the basic neuropsychological data collected for JL, GC, and FM when they initially presented. In all three patients there was a discrepancy between Verbal and Performance IQ (in favour of the latter) as measured using the Wechsler Adult Intelligence Scale–Revised (WAIS–R,

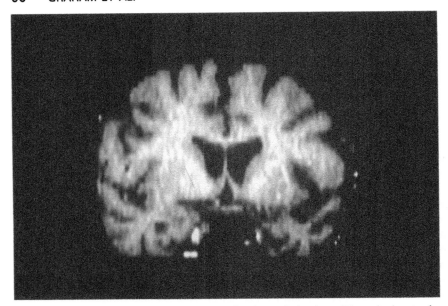

FIG. 5.2.   GC's MRI scan from June 1994 (coronally orientated) showing striking, selective atrophy
to the left infero-temporal gyri with preservation of the hippocampal formation.

Wechsler, 1981). This discrepancy was particularly noticeable in GC, and
results from impairments on the Vocabulary, Information, and Similarities subtests, which depend on knowledge of word meaning. By contrast, all three
patients' performance on Arithmetic, and on most Performance sub-tests was
substantially better. Likewise, on tests of visuo-spatial ability (copy of the
complex Rey Figure, Osterrieth, 1944) and non-verbal problem solving
(Raven's Coloured Progressive Matrices, Raven, 1962) their performance was
normal (see Fig. 5.3 for GC's copy of the Rey Figure). On a test of face
matching ability (Benton, Hamsher, Varney, & Spreen, 1983), JL and FM
showed no significant decrement, but GC performed slightly below the control
range. To test the comprehension of syntactic structures we administered the
80-item Test for the Reception of Grammar (TROG, Bishop, 1989) where
subjects are asked to point to the correct picture in response to progressively
more complex sentences (e.g. "The box is above the pen"; "The box but not the
chair is red") in which the major vocabulary items (nouns, verbs, and
adjectives) remain simple, high-frequency words even in the most syntactically
complicated sentences. While JL and FM showed no significant decrement on
this test, GC was mildly impaired, making eight errors (Controls: 1.3 ± 1.8). On
tests of episodic and working memory, there was no obvious impairment on
digit span, but the three patients showed variable performance on the delayed
recall of the Rey Figure and the Warrington Recognition Memory Test

Original Rey Figure (Osterrieth, 1944)

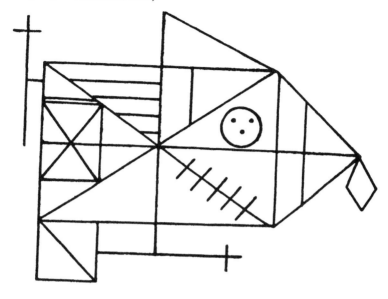

GC's Copy of the Rey Figure (2/2/93)

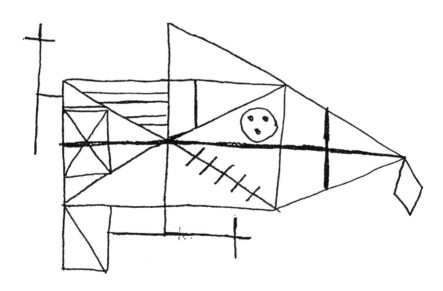

FIG. 5.3. GC's copy of the complex Rey Figure in February 1993 (Osterrieth, 1944).

TABLE 5.1
Summary of Neuropsychological Data (at Time of Initial Presentation)
on JL, GC, and FM

Test	JL	GC	FM	Controls n=24 mean (sd)
WAIS (scaled scores)—Information	2	4	4	
Vocabulary	1	6	5	
Arithmetic	11	9	9	
Similarities	1	4	5	
Picture Completion	4	11	6	
Block Design	9	12	8	
Digit Symbol	8	13	11	
WAIS—Verbal IQ	76	79	76	
WAIS—Performance IQ	85	117	98	
Visuoperceptual/Problem-Solving				
Rey Figure Copy (36)	34	36	31	34.0 (2.9)
Benton's Face Recognition Test (54)	50	38	42	41–54*
Raven's Coloured Matrices (36)	29	32	29	25 (50%ile)*
Language				
TROG (80)	76	72	76	78.8 (1.8)
Letter Fluency (F, A, and S)	14	14	23	44.6 (10.2)
Episodic/Working Memory				
Rey Figure—delayed recall (36)	16	18	5	15.2 (7,4)
WRMT Faces (50)	27	30	43	44 (3.8)
Digit Span Forwards	7	6	6	6.8 (1.0)
Digit Span Backwards	4	5	4	5 4.7 (1.2)
Semantic Memory				
Boston Naming Test (60)	10	8	6	55.8 (2.6)*
Pyramids and Palmtrees Test—3 pictures (52)	36	47	42	51.2 (1.4)
PALPA: Spoken WPM (40)	30	34	35	38.9 (2.2)
Category Fluency (animals)	10	6	3	17.5 (3.9)

WAIS = Wechsler Adult Intelligence Scale–Revised (Wechsler, 1981); WRMT = Warrington Recognition Memory Test (Warrington, 1984); TROG = Test for the Reception of Grammar (Bishop, 1989). Figures in brackets beside the tests indicate maximum possible scores. * = Original test norms for age-matched control subjects. The other norms for controls are from Hodges and Patterson (1995).

(Warrington, 1984). JL and GC showed normal performance on delayed recall of the Rey Figure, but noticeable impairment on the Faces version of the Warrington Recognition Memory Test. FM showed the opposite pattern of performance (normal recognition of unfamiliar faces, yet impaired recall of the Rey Figure).

There is no doubt that GC had a form of progressive aphasia, and the lack of phonological and syntactic errors in his spontaneous speech would seem to exclude the nonfluent form. We are left, therefore, with the question of whether his anomia (apparent on a range of tasks and in spontaneous conversation) reflects a breakdown in semantic memory (i.e. a case of semantic dementia, like JL) or rather, as in the case of FM, a kind of functional disconnection between the semantic and phonological systems. We (and many, though by no means all, other researchers) assume that semantic memory is an amodal system—that is, that largely the same base of conceptual knowledge about an object like a tiger is activated by seeing a picture of a tiger and by hearing or seeing the word tiger (Farah & McClelland, 1991; Vandenberghe et al., 1996). On this assumption, one would expect a deterioration in semantic memory itself to disrupt performance requiring conceptual knowledge across the board, whether the input to the system is a word or a picture and whether the response required is speech or some non-verbal action. This was true for JL; what about GC? The first data gathered from GC concerning the status of word and object comprehension were rather conflicting: although he showed impaired performance on word–picture matching, the degree of deficit was relatively mild in relation to his severe anomia. Moreover, on the three-picture version of the Pyramids and Palmtrees test his performance was only just below that of controls (see Table 5.1). In FM, the most revealing observations had come from the *longitudinal* assessment of her performance on naming and comprehension tasks. In an attempt to determine the nature of GC's word-finding difficulties, we shall now consider his performance on a range of tasks over time. We begin with the general picture (data from naming, reading, episodic memory, etc.) and then we shall consider some more specific results, from a task comparing words and pictures, to address the nature of GC's deficit.

GC'S LONGITUDINAL NEUROPSYCHOLOGICAL DATA

Word Production

The most profound symptom of both semantic dementia and progressive pure anomia is word-finding difficulty. These patients have little impairment of syntax and phonology, but their spontaneous speech is strikingly devoid of content words and often contains word-finding pauses. GC was given the

Cookie Theft picture description (part of the Boston Diagnostic Aphasia Examination, Goodglass & Kaplan, 1983), in which the subject is asked to describe, in as much detail as possible, a picture (which is set in a kitchen and comprises a woman washing up dishes, and two children conspiring to steal some cookies from a jar). GC managed to convey a reasonable amount of information about the picture and to produce a number of high-frequency nouns (girl, dishes, tree, cups etc.). On the other hand, there were a large number of word-finding pauses, as well as clear failures to retrieve a specific target word (e.g. he could not produce the word "sink" and had to settle for "the, eh … water system here").

Cookie Theft (May 1993)
Okay, looks like the kitchen, and there's a girl and a boy, and a mother and they're getting, eh … some cookies out of the, eh … jar here, and the boy's falling over from standing up too high and the girl looks like she's keeping quiet, don't tell your mother and the mother's washing … dishes and the water's over running out of the, eh … water system here. The window's open, eh … look's like the … eh … tree outside and the other part of the house is to the left with the window and eh … there's a couple of cups here she's already cleaned, washed and other than that, eh … she's standing on one leg with her other leg behind her. She has a dress on and she has a … eh … thing to, to, wash the, a eh … piece, a piece of that could be paper or, eh … something to water the, eh … dish with. Other than that there's, there's … eh … some doors down below here in the, eh … kitchen … down below and there's the floor. About all I can see.
KG: Is there anything else you want to say?
GC: Well I don't know what else to say, the little girl has, has, has eh … clothes on, shoes on and, eh … the boy has eh … pants on, and he has a little shirt on, and he also has eh … shoes on. Mother has shoes on … that's about all I could tell you.

Approximately a year later (mid-1994), GC's speech had become more impoverished. The amount of information he produced was significantly less (for example, in a conversation about tasks that he had been finding difficult at work, he did not provide any specific examples), the number of content words had been reduced (e.g. he talked about his parachuting by saying that, "I was one of the, the ones that fly around and jump out, you know") and there was an increase in the number of word-finding pauses. It is notable that GC rarely made any semantic or phonological errors.

The more quantitative tests of language, such as picture naming, support the conclusions from analyses of GC's spontaneous speech. His picture naming ability was moderately to severely impaired when he was first tested (118/260 items correct on the Snodgrass & Vanderwart (1980) corpus; 8/60 on the Boston Naming Test, Kaplan, Goodglass, & Weintraub, 1983), and continued to decline thereafter (5/60 on the BNT in October 1994) (see Table 5.2).

TABLE 5.2
A Summary of GC's Longitudinal Performance on a Range of
Neuropsychological Tests

Test	Time 1 (2/93)	Time 2 (10/94)	Time 3 (6/95)	Controls n=24 mean (sd)
Mini Mental State Examination (30)	27	20	20	29.2 (1.0)
WAIS (scaled scores)—Information	4	2	2	
Vocabulary	6	4	4	
Arithmetic	9	5	6	
Similarities	4	5	5	
Picture Completion	11	13	13	
Block Design	12	14	13	
Digit Symbol	13	11	10	
Object Assembly	12	12	12	
WAIS—Verbal IQ	79	72	71	
WAIS—Performance IQ	117	111	111	
WAIS—Full IQ	92	87	87	
Visuo-perceptual/Problem-solving				
Rey Figure Copy (36)	36	36	33	34.0 (2.9)
Benton's Face Recognition Test (54)	38	44	44	41–54*
Raven's Coloured Matrices (36)	32	33	NT	25(50 %ile)*
Language				
TROG (80)	72	72	62	78.8 (1.8)
Letter Fluency (F, A, and S)	14	21	13	44.6 (10.2)
Episodic/Working Memory				
Rey Figure—Immediate recall (36)	22	5.5	0	
Rey Figure—Delayed recall—45min (36)	18	8.5	0	15.2 (7.4)
WRMT—Faces (50)	30	28	NT	44 (3.8)
WRMT—Words (50)	32	26	NT	47 (2.8)
Digit Span Forwards	6	6	6	6.8 (1.0)
Digit Span Backwards	5	5	6	4.7 (1.2)
Word Span	3/4	4	2	NT
Semantic Memory				
Boston Naming Test (60)	8	5	NT	55.8 (2.6)*
Pyramids and Palmtrees Test—3 pictures (52)	47	42	42	51.2 (1.4)
PALPA: Spoken WPM (40)	34	27	21	38.9 (2.2)
PALPA: Written WPM (40)	31	28	NT	39.5 (1.0)*
PALPA: Auditory Synonym Judgement (60)	46	28	NT	NT
PALPA: Written Synonym Judgement (60)	41	29	NT	NT
Category Fluency (animals)	6	4	2	17.5 (3.9)

For abbreviations see the legend for Table 5.1.

He was even more severely impaired when asked to produce the name of an item from an appropriate description (i.e. "a small green animal which leaps around ponds"), scoring zero out of 48 items.

In contrast to GC's deterioration on semantically based tests of language production, his performance on letter fluency, in which subjects are asked to produce as many words (excluding proper nouns) as they can in one minute beginning with each of three letters (F, A, S), showed no deterioration over the 27 months of testing: although his performance on this test was somewhat variable, he produced a total of 14 items in February 1993 and 13 in June 1995. On category fluency, however, GC's score fell from six to two animals over the same period, and in June 1995, he failed to produce any correct responses for three other more specific animal categories (birds, sea creatures, and dogs). This contrast between category fluency, which depends on activation of semantic representations, and letter fluency, which may access more directly the phonological output lexicon, has been noted in other patients with breakdown in semantic memory (Hodges & Patterson, 1996; Rosser & Hodges, 1994). In May 1994, GC was also unable to produce descriptions of a number of common animals and objects; this is discussed in more detail later.

Word Comprehension

GC initially showed mild-to-moderate impairment on tests of word comprehension (word–picture matching and synonym judgement etc.) and, on follow-up over 28 months, his performance deteriorated on all such tests (see Table 5.2 and Fig. 5.4). His performance on a within-category word–picture matching test (selecting one of eight related exemplars to match a spoken word) had also fallen to a very low level: GC correctly pointed to 23/48 items (48%), whereas controls score flawlessly on this task.

It should be noted that GC has more recently started to show additional problems with syntactic comprehension, as measured by the Test for the Reception of Grammar (Bishop, 1989), on which his performance dropped from 72/80 in February 1993 to 62/80 in June 1995.

Non-verbal Semantic Tasks

On non-verbal tests of semantic memory, GC was also impaired. For example, when asked to colour-in black-and-white line drawings of common objects, he scored 60% in May 1993, a score that was below normal limits (75–95%). His drawing from memory was exceptionally poor at this time: out of 20 items, only 5 were judged by "blind" raters as representative of the target item (see Fig. 5.5), and he failed to produce any response at all for 8 of the 20 items. The fact that GC was able to copy complex geometric figures almost flawlessly excludes a significant visuo-spatial or praxic deficit.

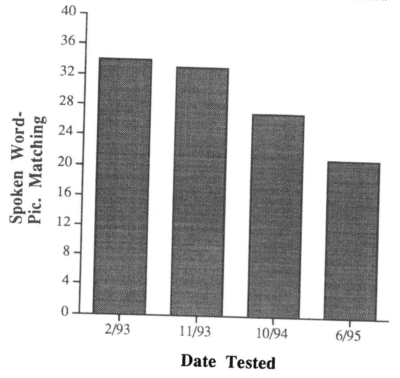

FIG. 5.4. GC's performance on the spoken word–picture matching test from the PALPA (Kay et al., 1992) over time (from February 1993 to June 1995).

Reading

The majority of patients with progressive fluent aphasia are surface dyslexic (see for example Parkin, 1993; Patterson & Hodges, 1992). In pure surface dyslexia, patients retain normal ability to read aloud words with regular spelling-to-sound correspondences (HINT, FLINT etc.), but make a significant number of errors when asked to read words with irregular spelling-to-sound correspondences, predominantly regularisation errors (e.g. PINT pronounced to rhyme with HINT) (Marshall & Newcombe, 1973). In line with this pattern, GC was unable to read virtually any of the low-frequency irregular words used in the National Adult Reading Test of Nelson (1982) e.g. THYME, DEBT, BOUQUET etc. Although he showed a significant discrepancy between regular and exception words, like JL (but not FM who was initially normal on regular words) GC cannot be described as having a pure surface dyslexia. For example, on the reading test from the PALPA (Kay et al., 1992), he correctly read 73% of

Drawing from memory (elephant, sock, and penguin)

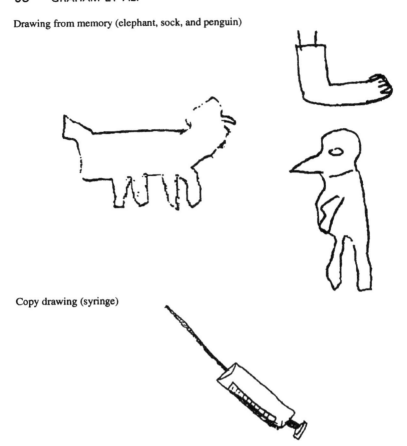

Copy drawing (syringe)

FIG. 5.5.   GC's drawing from memory of an elephant, sock, and penguin, and his copy drawing of a black-and-white line drawing of a syringe.

the regular words and 50% of the frequency-matched exception words. By June 1995, his scores had fallen to 53% and 43% correct for the regular and exception words, respectively. On another reading task composed of 53 frequency- and length-matched pairs of regular and exception, words, GC made 7 errors when reading the regular words, compared with 24 errors when reading the exception words. All the errors were for medium- and low-frequency target items (Graham et al., 1994). Also like JL, GC showed a further impairment to nonword reading (58% correct), consistent with his increasing difficulty with regular, as well as exception, word reading. His nonword reading was also affected by length: he made more errors on items comprising six letters compared with nonwords comprising three letters.

Episodic Memory

At first, GC showed no obvious deficit in either short-term/working memory (his digit span remained normal over the past two years) or episodic memory. He was well orientated in time and place, and when tested six months after his initial presentation he was able to provide examples of recent personal events. For example, he was asked to produce an episode from the past related to the word "successful" (an example from a cued autobiographical test based on the Galton-Crovitz technique, Crovitz & Schiffman, 1974), and responded:

GC: Successful. Well, successful, I feel successful when I get things done and finished up and everything works okay, so it doesn't eh ... there's no problems. Just like out back there I painted all the, the eh ... things out there and I fixed them all up. I put new screws on them and some new wood parts on and I made all the paints and it was all successful.
KG: When was that?
GC: I did that a month ago.

He also seemed competent in prospective memory. When asked, in May 1993, about his church meetings, he responded:

GC: Well actually, it's eh ... it's the meeting that we eh ... set up eh ... for the kids, eh ... over there on different things. In fact, there's the latest one is going to be 6.30 June 21st, the committee eh ... we're going to be doing some salad. I'm going to take some salad over there.

The results from the Galton-Crovitz test show that, at least in May 1993, GC was able to produce autobiographical memories from the past, most of which were episodes specific in time and place. Interestingly, virtually all of the events were from the very recent past (i.e. the last three months). This pattern suggests that, like other patients with focal atrophy to the temporal neocortex, GC may have better preservation of recent memories than distant memories (Graham & Hodges, 1997).

On the basis of more conventional tests of episodic memory, however, it would be difficult to argue for the integrity of GC's anterograde memory. For example, while his copy of the Rey Figure (Osterrieth, 1944) has shown little deterioration over the past two years, immediate and delayed recall of the Rey have deteriorated quite dramatically, to the extent that he scored zero on both recall components in June 1995[1]. His performance on other tests of memory, such as the Warrington Recognition Memory Test (Warrington, 1984) where the subject is shown 50 words (or faces) and later asked to

---

[1]More recent testing (February 1996), revealed improved performance on this test (immediate recall = 11 and delayed recall = 7).

identify which (from pairs of stimuli) had been seen previously, also dropped from poor in February 1993 to chance level in October 1994 (see Table 5.2).

In summary, while GC was unimpaired on non-verbal episodic memory when he was initially tested and for sometime into his illness, his ability to establish new memories appears to have deteriorated since then. This result suggests that GC may now be starting to show more generalised cognitive problems.

Problem-solving and Visuo-spatial Abilities

Briefly, GC has shown no significant deterioration on any of the tests used to measure non-verbal problem-solving ability (e.g. Raven's Coloured Progressive Matrices, Raven, 1962) or visuo-spatial skills (e.g. the Rey Copy; the visuo-spatial components of the WAIS–R such as Block Design and Picture Assembly [Wechsler, 1981], and the Benton Face Recognition Test [Benton et al., 1983]). This is in contrast to his decline on the Arithmetic, Vocabulary and Information "Verbal" sub-tests of the WAIS–R. The preservation of these non-verbal cognitive skills has also been observed in other reported cases of progressive fluent aphasia, and both JL and FM showed similarly intact performance on these types of test.

MODALITY-SPECIFIC DIFFERENCES IN GC'S PERFORMANCE: PICTURES VS WORDS

At his first evaluation, GC attained only slightly abnormal performance (47/52) on the three-picture version of the Pyramids and Palmtrees test (Howard & Patterson, 1992); two years later, his score had declined somewhat, to 42 (81%). On the corresponding three-word version of this test, however, he showed a much more profound impairment, scoring 30/52 (58%) in June 1995. In other words, there has been a more dramatic decline on word-based semantic tasks than on picture-based tests; but it is not obvious from this simple fact that the most appropriate interpretation is a modality-specific pattern of semantic impairment. The relationship between the surface properties of an object name and the nature of the object to which it refers is completely arbitrary; the name in isolation gives away no conceptual information "for free". A picture of the object, on the other hand, provides or affords a substantial amount of information about the type of thing represented, even if the specific object itself is not fully recognised or comprehended. Thus, while a pattern like GC's of greater success with picture- than word-based semantic tests might suggest that different conceptual knowledge bases are activated by the two types of stimulus materials (as argued by Warrington & McCarthy, 1994), it is also possible that this differential success merely reflects the contrasting richness of information in the two stimulus types themselves (Caramazza, Hillis, Rapp, &

Romani, 1990). In order to explore this issue in somewhat more detail, we administered a definitions test, in which GC was asked to describe a number of common objects (n=48, including animals and manmade items), in response both to spoken words and to the corresponding line drawings from the Snodgrass and Vanderwart (1980) corpus. These definitions were assessed on several different occasions, so that the same item was never tested in both modalities on the same day.

GC's definitions, although strikingly impoverished from both modalities, were qualitatively rather different for words and pictures. For example, to the spoken word "tiger", GC could only respond "Animal, four legs". When given the picture of a tiger, he produced: "Another animal. Another four legs, two ears, two eyes, a nose, a mouth. It strictly walks, it doesn't go in the water. Its legs are very long, it also has parts on its legs."

Similarly, to the spoken word "bicycle", GC said only: "Something you ride with, something you move your legs with, up and down." His response when given the picture of the bicycle, however, was: "Bicycle, it has two places you can put your feet on the bottom and spread back and forth to keep it going forward, you can also stop it. There's two places up on top, one for each side your hands can put on. There's a place you can sit on. Other than that you can go back and forth."

These examples (and further ones given in Table 5.3) demonstrate that GC's definitions in response to spoken words were particularly sparse, whereas he apparently generated more information in response to the corresponding pictures. As indicated earlier, however, we must ask the following question with regard to this contrast in the quality and detail of the information produced in the two versions of the definitions task: do pictures make contact with a different (and, in GC's case, more intact) set of semantic knowledge from that activated by words? Or is it rather the case that much of what GC was able to say about pictures could be either directly seen in, or else inferred from, the line drawing? Definitions are a rich and unstructured type of response, which can be scored in various ways (see for example Hodges, Patterson, Graham, & Dawson, 1996); but in order to address this specific question, we simply assigned each of GC's 96 definitions (48 for the objects as names, 48 for the same objects as line drawings) to one of the following four categories:

1. Don't know.
2. Superordinate only: GC's only response was to indicate the broad superordinate category to which the object belongs (e.g. "it's an animal" or "a musical thing", etc.).
3. Generic information only: by this we refer to either (a) (for responses to pictures) information directly visible in the picture (e.g. to the picture of a crocodile: "it's kind of long and has four legs"), or (b) (for responses to either

TABLE 5.3
Examples of GC's Definitions from Spoken Words and Pictures
(Black-and-White Line Drawing)

Item	Definition (Spoken Word)	Definition (Picture)
Crocodile	Animal.	It's kind of long and it has four legs and he swims in the water. And he has a big mouth and two small eyes. Four pieces of feet.
Fox	Animal, has four feet, two ears, two eyes.	A large animal, and it has a very long, eh, in the back there, it has four legs, two ears, two eyes, he has a piece in his mouth. Other than that he just walks, he doesn't fly or swim or anything, mostly he just walks with his four legs.
Lobster	Animal.	It's another animal, it flies around and it strictly all flies and it's got two large arms up front there and it has two long ears. There's some things on the right and left of the body that will scratch your arms too, it's kind of heavy.
Hen	Can't remember what a hen is.	Another animal and it has two legs, two eyes, one mouth, it also has two portions on the side that she could fly. They could fly up and down and around. It's a bird, it could fly up and down and around other than that they don't go in the water, they strictly fly around and sit up in the trees and things.
Violin	Don't know.	That's an item that you put in your arms and start to scratch it back and forth, there's a place right at the bottom there that you could flip it back and forth, it creates noise. There's also one, one let me see, there's, four lines that could be scratched back and forth.
Airplane	Something you fly in, you can fly all over the country or all over the world.	It's an airplane and it flies up and back it has two large areas in front and two smaller in back and there's a place in front there that they look outside, there's also little places one each side of the airplane. It flies up and down.
Desk	Thing that you keep your papers on and also in the drawers. Keep your paper and different things.	It looks like it has seven places to open. Other than that there is four parts on the bottom of it, there is also a place you can write on it, also you can put things inside each one of these places here. You can put telephones on top of it and you keep things inside.
Drum	You could play it, bang on.	That's something that you would play by touching on top, making a noise setting things up, it would be eh, to make a, other than that it's very big too.

words or pictures) information that is generally characteristic of the *kind* of thing named or pictured without indicating any distinctive knowledge about the specific instance. For example, to the spoken name "fox", GC said "animal, has four feet, two ears, two eyes", which is true of a very large number of animals; to the picture of a hen, GC responded "it has two portions on the side so that she could fly", which is true of the majority of birds.

4. Specific information: here we include information that goes beyond what is obvious from the picture and furthermore that is distinctively characteristic of the object in question, e.g. that cows give milk and hens lay eggs and crocodiles are dangerous, that drums are played by banging on them, that desks are used to write on or keep papers in, and so on.

The results of this analysis are presented in Fig. 5.6, which indicates the following two important outcomes of comparing the modalities of stimulus presentation. First of all, GC's performance in the two modalities differed in that there were a number of instances for word stimuli where he either offered no information at all about the object named or gave only the word's very general category; by contrast, these "don't know" and superordinate-only responses were never produced for picture stimuli. Second, however, and of particular note: in those cases where GC was able to say something about an object beyond its superordinate class, performance in the two modalities was strikingly similar. That is, although of course there were many more pictures than words where GC's definition had some substance (because virtually no pictures yielded don't-know or superordinate-only responses), the two modalities yielded a very similar balance between responses containing something specifically identifying about the object and cases where the only available information was generic. So, for pictures as well as words, many of GC's definitions contained only information obtainable or inferable from the picture itself and lacked any information that would have to be activated from concept-specific semantics.

Note that the kind of information that we have termed generic will typically apply to a given object, but can also be erroneous. Thus, for example, GC's assertion that the picture of a lobster was "an animal that flies around" presumably indicates that he had interpreted the lobster's claws as wings. His comment on the picture of the hen ("it sits up in trees") suggests that he recognised the hen as a bird and inferred from his generic bird-knowledge that the hen would sit in trees; but that he may not, even from the picture, have been able to activate any hen-specific knowledge.

GC's performance on the definitions task as a whole, plus some more detailed characteristics summarised earlier, suggest the following interpretation. Across the board, GC's descriptions of these familiar objects were strikingly impoverished; this is consistent with a deficit of semantic, conceptual knowledge. Despite the apparent superiority in the extent and

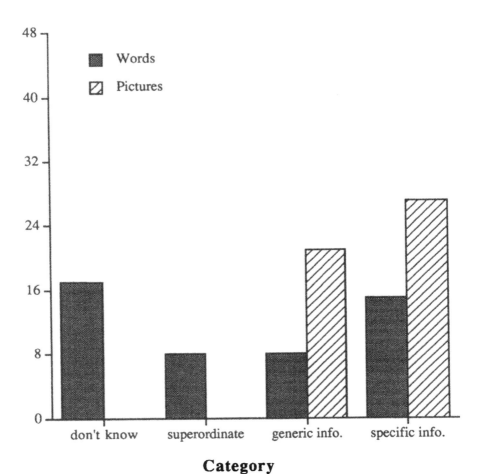

Category

FIG. 5.6.   Categorisation of GC's definitions from a spoken word and from a black-and-white line drawing. There were four categories: (1) don't know, (2) superordinate only (e.g. "animal", "its a musical thing" etc.), (3) generic information only (e.g. information that is characteristic of the *kind* of thing named or pictured, for example, many land animals have four legs, or, in the case of pictures, information directly visible from the drawing), (4) specific information (e.g. information that is distinctively characteristic of the object—drums are played by banging on them; hens lay eggs).

quality of his responses to pictures as compared to word stimuli, almost all of the picture advantage can be explained in terms of differential information afforded by the stimuli themselves. If GC still had some reasonably intact degree of knowledge about a concept (such as a desk or an airplane; see the examples of his definitions to these in Table 5.3), then his definition to both word and picture contained some concept-specific information; and anything extra that he said in response to the picture was largely attributable to information available in the line drawing. If his semantic knowledge about a concept had significantly deteriorated (as for lobster or hen), then he could say little in response to the spoken name because the word yields so few clues to the nature of the object; but his more extensive responses to the corresponding pictures give only a spurious sense that the picture has contacted a more detailed knowledge base than the word, because most of the information that he offered was limited to features that are visible in, or inferable from, the pictures. There is nothing in these results that seems to demand an interpretation of modality-specific semantic knowledge. More to the point for an understanding of GC, we conclude from these results that, despite GC's apparently disproportionate impairment on word-based tests, his deficit is not limited to word processing but is best characterised as progressive aphasia resulting from a central semantic deterioration.

DISCUSSION

Patients with primary progressive aphasia can have one of (at least) three patterns of deficit: (a) a breakdown to the syntactic and phonological processes of language: this is progressive nonfluent aphasia; (b) a deterioration of semantic memory affecting language perhaps most blatantly but other cognitive abilities that rely on semantic memory as well: this is semantic dementia, the usual pattern seen in progressive fluent aphasia; and (c) a disruption of communication between semantic memory and phonology: this is progressive pure anomia, another variety of fluent aphasia. Given the fluency of GC's speech, the relative preservation of his syntactic comprehension and the lack of phonological errors in his spontaneous speech, it seems clear that GC does not have a progressive nonfluent aphasia. The question of his semantic memory impairment is a little more complex: at least initially, there was a marked discrepancy between his profoundly impaired ability to find words (both in spontaneous speech and on formal tests of picture naming, naming to description, and category fluency) and his much milder deficit on tests of semantic memory that do not involve speech production (especially object-based semantic tasks such as the Pyramids and Palmtrees Test). The contrast between GC's severely abnormal category fluency and his more successful (though far from normal) letter fluency suggests that his word production ability was particularly stressed by tasks in which the phonological word form must be activated by a semantic specification.

Although picture naming and other word production tasks seem to be particularly sensitive to deterioration of semantic knowledge, we acknowledge that GC's semantic impairment may not have been the only factor contributing to his anomia. That is, GC's central semantic deficit may have been exacerbated by a further deficit in communication between semantic and phonological representations. Longitudinal testing, however, does not support the hypothesis that the locus of GC's anomia, like that of FM, was *primarily* this semantic→phonological interface. One of the most striking reasons for considering FM to be uniquely different from patients with semantic dementia was the fact that, although her performance on some semantic tests was mildly impaired on initial testing, these scores showed no noticeable decline over three years during which she was extensively investigated. Although GC's semantic deterioration has been much slower than that seen in some other reported patients with semantic dementia (e.g. Hodges et al., 1994, 1995), he has in fact declined on all administered tests of semantic memory (see Table 5.2 and Fig. 5.4).

We turn now, briefly, to GC's pattern of performance on tests of semantic memory and its potential implications for models of semantic memory. Modality of presentation (i.e. words vs pictures) certainly influenced both GC's quantitative scores on tests like Pyramids and Palm Trees and the qualitative nature of his responses on the definitions task. One main theoretical division in models of semantic memory is between those that propose modality-specific subsets of knowledge, that is to say separate visually and verbally based semantic systems (Shallice, 1987; Warrington & McCarthy, 1994), and those that consider conceptual knowledge to be represented in an essentially amodal network which is accessed from a number of sensory channels (Caramazza et al., 1990; Chertkow, Bub, & Caplan, 1992; Riddoch, Humphreys, Coltheart, & Funnell, 1988). Does GC's apparently consistent advantage for performance with pictures relative to words argue, as face validity might suggest, for the former type of account? As indicated in our discussion of GC's definitions, we do not consider such a conclusion to be warranted. More detailed analyses of GC and other patients with degraded semantic memory will obviously be required before any coherent account can emerge from a complex set of findings; but our interim interpretation is that GC's modality discrepancy can be explained by an account in which both words and pictures activate more or less the same central conceptual representations. The apparent picture superiority is explained in terms of information inherent in or afforded by the pictures that cannot be obtained from word forms; and our confidence that GC was relying to a large extent on such "affordances" in his picture definitions is increased by the fact that he made a number of errors on just such grounds. A picture of a bird-like animal "affords" the general inference that the creature can fly and sits in trees, an inference that is correct for most birds but wrong for a few specific instances of this category. GC's definition of the *hen* picture contained the "fact" that it sits in trees, which to us suggests reliance on the general affordance rather than retrieval of a specific semantic feature for *hen*.

Our claim that GC's modality-specific *performance* does not require a modality-specific *theory* is not tantamount to a claim that the post-stimulus processing of words and pictures is identical. In highly connected, interactive networks of the sort that we imagine to be responsible for semantic processing, differences at one level of the system (such as those between verbal and pictorial input) can have pervasive effects at other levels (see Plaut & Shallice, 1993, for a relevant discussion). Therefore, if some concepts are initially acquired and/or typically encountered mainly by interacting with the objects themselves whereas other object concepts are mainly encountered from verbal input, then one might expect some significant interactions between categories of concept and modality of presentation (Farah & McClelland, 1991). Furthermore, it is surely not the case that we activate all of our semantic knowledge about a given concept on every occasion on which we encounter it; and the specific subset of semantic features activated may vary not only from one occasion and context to another, but also as a function of mode of input. Thus, even for semantic knowledge that is frequently accessed both by real objects and words, the particular features of a given object that are activated by hearing its name and by seeing an instance of it may have some fairly consistent distributional differences. It may be easier for theorists to think and talk about these subtle differences by postulating separate systems; but that is not necessarily a reliable guide to the way in which information is represented in the brain.

If we assume that the principal deficit in GC is, indeed, a breakdown in semantic memory, then the site of pathology might inform us about the neural basis of this most fundamental of cognitive abilities. Although work on semantic memory is still in its infancy, there is accruing evidence that regions of the temporal lobe play a critical role. In other patients with semantic dementia, the most consistently involved region has been the left infero-lateral temporal neocortex (Breedin, Saffran, & Coslett, 1994; Hodges et al., 1992a; Hodges & Patterson, 1996; Parkin, 1993; Patterson & Hodges, 1995); some patients have bilateral pathology while others exhibit only left-sided cortical atrophy. The medial temporal lobe complex (hippocampus, parahippocampal gyrus, subiculum etc.) is important for the encoding and storage of recently acquired episodic memories, and it appears that closely connected neocortical temporal regions may act as the storage site for very long-term information, including semantic memory. There are also hints that parallel right-sided temporal lobe structures are specialised for person-based, rather than general, semantic information (Evans, Heggs, Antoun, & Hodges, 1995). The key role assigned to this infero-temporal region in human semantic memory accords with primate research, which has shown that the ventral stream of high-level visual information destined for the antero-infero temporal lobe carries information concerned with object identification and recognition (Ungerleider & Mishkin, 1982).

ACKNOWLEDGEMENTS

We would like to thank the patients and control subjects included in this paper for their time and patience, and S.T.-DeKosky, MD for allowing the detailed evaluation of GC. This research was supported by a MRC Project Grant and a Wellcome Trust Grant to JRH. JTB received support from a Research Scientist Development Award (K02-MH0177) and the Alzheimer's Disease Research Center (AG05133).

REFERENCES

Barbarotto, R., Capitani, E., Spinnler, H., & Trivelli, C. (1995). Slowly progressive semantic impairment with category specificity. *Neurocase, 1*, 107–119.

Benton, A.L., Hamsher, K. deS., Varney, N.R., & Spreen, O. (1983). *Contributions to neuropsychological assessment*, New York: Oxford University Press.

Bishop, D.V.M. (1989). *Test for the Reception of Grammar* (2nd Edn.). Manchester, UK: Author (available from the Department of Psychology, University of Manchester, Manchester, UK).

Breedin, S., Saffran, E., & Coslett, B. (1994). Reversal of the concreteness effect in a patient with semantic dementia. *Cognitive Neuropsychology, 11*, 617–660.

Caramazza, A., Hillis, A.E., Rapp, B.C., & Romani, C. (1990). The multiple semantics hypothesis: Multiple confusions? *Cognitive Neuropsychology, 7*, 161–189.

Caselli, R.J., Jack, C.R., Petersen, R.C., Wahner, H.W., & Yanagihara, T. (1992). Asymmetric cortical degenerative syndromes: Clinical and radiologic correlations. *Neurology, 42*, 1462–1468.

Chertkow, H., Bub, D., & Caplan, D. (1992). Constraining theories of semantic memory processing: Evidence from dementia. *Cognitive Neuropsychology, 9*, 327–365.

Croot, K., Patterson, K., & Hodges, J.R. (in press). Single-word production in nonfluent progressive aphasia. *Brain and Language*.

Crovitz, H.F., & Schiffman, H. (1974). Frequency of episodic memories as a function of their age. *Bulletin of the Psychonomic Society, 4*, 517–518.

Evans, J.J., Heggs, A.J., Antoun, N., & Hodges, J.R. (1995). Progressive prosopagnosia associated with selective right temporal lobe atrophy: A new syndrome? *Brain, 118*, 1–13.

Farah, M.J., & McClelland, J.L. (1991). A computational model of semantic memory impairment: Modality specificity and emergent category specificity. *Journal of Experimental Psychology: General, 20*, 339–357.

Goodglass, H., & Kaplan, E. (1983). *The assessment of aphasia and related disorders* (2nd Edn.). Philadelphia: Lea & Febiger.

Graham, K., Patterson, K., & Hodges, J.R. (1995). Progressive pure anomia: Insufficient activation of phonology by meaning. *Neurocase, 1*, 25–38.

Graham, K.S., & Hodges, J.R. (1997). Differentiating the roles of the hippocampal system and the neocortex in long-term memory storage: Evidence from the study of semantic dementia and Alzheimer's disease, *Neuropsychology: 11*, 77–89.

Graham, K.S., Hodges, J.R., & Patterson, K. (1994). The relationship between comprehension and oral reading in progressive fluent aphasia. *Neuropsychologia, 32,* 299–316.

Hodges, J.R., Graham, N.E., & Patterson, K. (1995). Charting the progression in semantic dementia: Implications for the organisation of semantic memory. *Memory, 3/4,* 463–495.

Hodges, J.R., & Patterson, K. (1995). Is semantic memory consistently impaired early in the course of Alzheimer's disease? Neuroanatomical and diagnostic implications. *Neuropsychologia, 33,* 441–459.

Hodges, J.R., & Patterson, K. (1996). Non-fluent progressive aphasia and semantic dementia: A comparative neuropsychological study. *Journal of the International Neuropsychology Society.*

Hodges, J.R., Patterson, K., Graham, N., & Dawson, K. (1996). Naming and knowing in dementia of Alzheimer's Type. *Brain and Language, 54,* 302–325.

Hodges, J.R., Patterson, K., Oxbury, S., & Funnell, E. (1992a). Semantic dementia: Progressive fluent aphasia with temporal lobe atrophy. *Brain, 115,* 1783–1806.

Hodges, J.R., Patterson, K., & Tyler, L.K. (1994). Loss of semantic memory: Implications for the modularity of mind. *Cognitive Neuropsychology, 11*(5), 505–542.

Hodges, J.R., Salmon, D.P., & Butters, N. (1992b). Semantic memory impairment in Alzheimer's disease: Failure of access or degraded knowledge? *Neuropsychologia, 30,* 301–314.

Howard, D., & Patterson, K. (1992). *Pyramids and Palm Trees: A test of semantic access from pictures and words.* Bury St Edmunds, UK: Thames Valley Test Company.

Kaplan, E., Goodglass, H., & Weintraub, S. (1983). *Boston Naming Test.* Philadelphia: Lea & Febiger.

Karbe, H., Kertesz, A., & Polk, M. (1993). Profiles of language impairment in primary progressive aphasia. *Archives of Neurology, 50,* 193–201.

Kay, J., Lesser, R., & Coltheart, M. (1992). *Psycholinguistic assessment of language processing in aphasia.* Hove, UK: Lawrence Erlbaum Associates Ltd.

Marshall, J.C., & Newcombe, F. (1973). Patterns of paralexia: A psycholinguistic approach. *Journal of Psycholinguistic Research, 2,* 175–199.

Mesulam, M.M. (1982). Slowly progressive aphasia without generalised dementia. *Annals of Neurology, 11,* 592–598.

Mesulam, M.M., & Weintraub, S. (1992). Primary progressive aphasia. In F. Boller (Ed.), *Heterogeneity of Alzheimer's disease,* pp. 43–66. Berlin: Springer-Verlag.

Mingazzini, G. (1914). On aphasia due to atrophy of the cerebral convolutions. *Brain, 36,* 493–524.

Nelson, H.E. (1982). *The National Adult Reading Test (NART): Test Manual.* Windsor, UK: NFER-Nelson.

Osterrieth, P.A. (1944). Le test de copie d'une figure complexe: Contribution a l'étude de la perception et de la memoire. *Archives de Psychologies, Geneva, 30,* 205–220.

Parkin, A.J. (1993). Progressive aphasia without dementia due to focal left temporo-frontal hypometabolism—A clinical and cognitive neuropsychological analysis. *Brain and Language, 44,* 201–220.

Patterson, K., & Hodges, J.R. (1992). Deterioration of word-meaning: Implications for reading. *Neuropsychologia, 30,* 1025–1040.

Patterson, K., & Hodges, J.R. (1995). Disorders of semantic memory. In A.D. Baddeley, B.A. Wilson & F.N. Watts (Eds.), *Handbook of memory disorders,* pp. 167–186. Chichester, UK: John Wiley & Sons Ltd.

Pick, A. (1892). Uber die Beziehungen der senilen Hirnatrophie zur Aphasie. *Prager Medizinsche Wochenschrift, 17,* 165–167.

Plaut, D.C., & Shallice, T. (1993). Deep dyslexia: A case study of connectionist neuropsychology. *Cognitive Neuropsychology, 10,* 377–500.

Poeck, K., & Luzzatti, C. (1988). Slowly progressive aphasia in three patients: The problem of accompanying neuropsychological deficit. *Brain, 111,* 151–168.

Raven, J.C. (1962). *Coloured Progressive Matrices Sets A, AB, B.* London: H.K. Lewis.

Riddoch, M.J., Humphreys, G.W., Coltheart, M., & Funnell, E. (1988). Semantic systems or system? Neuropsychological evidence re-examined. *Cognitive Neuropsychology, 5,* 3–25.

Rosser, A., & Hodges, J.R. (1994). Initial letter and semantic category fluency in Alzheimer's disease, Huntington's disease and supranuclear palsy. *Journal of Neurology, Neurosurgery and Psychiatry, 57,* 1389–1394.

Scheltens, P., Ravid, R., & Kamphurst, W. (1994). Pathologic findings in a case of primary progressive aphasia. *Neurology, 44,* 279–282.

Shallice, T. (1987). Impairments of semantic processing: Multiple dissociations. In M. Coltheart, G. Sartori & R. Job (Eds.), *The cognitive neuropsychology of language,* pp. 111–127. Hove, UK: Lawrence Erlbaum Associates Ltd.

Snodgrass, J.G., & Vanderwart, M. (1980). A standardised set of 260 pictures: Norms for name agreement, familiarity and visual complexity. *Journal of Experimental Psychology: General, 6,* 174–215.

Snowden, J.S., Goulding, P.J., & Neary, D. (1989). Semantic dementia: A form of circumscribed cerebral atrophy. *Behavioural Neurology, 2,* 167–182.

Snowden, J..S., Neary, D., Mann, D.M.A., Goulding, P.J., & Testa, H.J. (1992). Progressive language disorder due to lobar atrophy. *Annals of Neurology, 31,* 174–183.

Tyler, L.K. (1992). *Spoken language comprehension: An experimental approach to disordered and normal processing.* Cambridge, MA: MIT Press.

Tyler, L.K., Moss, H.E., Patterson, K., & Hodges, J.R. (1997). The gradual deterioration of syntax and semantics in a patient with progressive aphasia. *Brain and Language, 56,* 426–476.

Tyrrell, P.J., Warrington, K.E., Frackowiak, R.S., & Rossor, M.N. (1990). Heterogeneity in progressive aphasia due to focal cortical atrophy. A clinical and PET study. *Brain, 113,* 1321–1336.

Warrington, E.K. (1984). *Recognition Memory Test.* Windsor, UK: NFER-Nelson.

Warrington, E.K., & McCarthy, R. (1994). Multiple meaning systems in the brain: A case for visual semantics. *Neuropsychologia, 32,* 1465–1473.

Wechsler, D. (1981). *WAIS–R manual.* New York: The Psychological Corporation.

Ungerleider, L.G., & Mishkin, M. (1982). Two cortical visual systems. In D.J. Ingle, M.A. Goodale & R.J.W. Mansfield (Eds.), *Analysis of visual behaviour,* pp. 549–586. Cambridge, MA: MIT Press.

Vandenberghe, R., Price, C., Wise, R.J.S., Josephs, O., & Frackowiak, R.S.J. (1996). Functional-anatomy of a common semantic system for words and pictures: *Nature, 383,* 254–256.

6 Impaired Recall and Preserved Recognition

J. Richard Hanley
University of Liverpool, UK

Ann D.M. Davies
University of Liverpool,
District Psychology Service, Wirral Community Healthcare, UK

INTRODUCTION

Traditionally, it has been assumed that patients who have problems in remembering events that have taken place since the time of their illness or accident perform badly on formal tests of memory regardless of whether performance is assessed by tests of recall or by tests of recognition (e.g. Warrington & Weislantz, 1970). In a recent review of 33 published papers in which patients with memory impairments had been administered Warrington's (1984) Recognition Memory test (RMT), however, Aggleton and Shaw (1996, p.57) concluded that there was "evidence of a systematic difference" in recognition performance. In the majority of cases, performance on tests of new learning was extremely poor on both recall and recognition. In some cases, however, it was clear that recognition memory was much less severely impaired than recall. In the last few years, along with our colleagues John Downes and Andrew Mayes, we have had the opportunity of working with one of the patients (ROB) that led Aggleton and Shaw to draw this conclusion. On the Warrington RMT for words, for instance, ROB scored 47/50 (controls mean = 44.8), yet her recall performance on the WMS–R (Wechsler, 1988) revealed a verbal memory quotient of 69, some 49 points below her Verbal IQ.

In this chapter, we will review some of the key comparisons between recall and recognition that we made in our original published report of ROB

(Hanley, Davies, Downes, & Mayes, 1994). We will also describe the results of some new experiments, conducted more recently, that have investigated her performance on different types of recognition memory test. This enables us to make some interesting comparisons between the performance of ROB and that of another recently published case, CB (Parkin, Yeomans, & Bindschaedler, 1994), who also shows a disproportionately strong recall of impairment.

CASE DETAILS

ROB suffered a ruptured anterior communicating artery aneurysm in 1990 when she was 42 years old At the time, she was working as a primary school teacher and living at home with her husband and children. The aneurysm was clipped in a surgical operation that was described as "routine" and ROB made a good physical recovery. CT scans taken a few months later indicated severe damage to the caudate nucleus in the left hemisphere, but no evidence of right hemisphere injury. Volumetric analysis of a sequence of MR scans confirmed this, and also revealed no evidence of any overall loss of volume in either the left frontal lobe or the hippocampus. The MR scans also showed some loss of volume at the anterior end of the thalamus in the left relative to the right hemisphere.

The results of neuropsychological testing were consistent with above average general intellectual functioning. On the WAIS–R (Wechsler, 1981), Verbal IQ was 118, and Performance IQ was 121. These figures were consistent with estimates of ROB's pre-morbid IQ (Nelson, 1982). Performance on written and spoken tests of language production and comprehension was excellent, as was performance on tests of imagery and famous face recognition.

Memory Function

A very different pattern was revealed when episodic memory function was examined. In the period immediately following her operation, ROB had shown evidence of confusion and confabulation. This was not surprising as confabulation during the early stages of recovery in ACoA patients is extremely common (DeLuca & Cicerone, 1991). For example, a diary that ROB kept while in hospital contained entries which made it clear that she believed she was back at teacher training college. When we tested her several months later, however, there was no sign of confabulation in either her diary entries or from her performance on a test of autobiographical memory (Robinson, 1976). Nevertheless, ROB had at this time returned to her teaching job in a part-time capacity, and was complaining of severe everyday memory problems that were making it difficult for her to function effectively either at home or at school. Her performance on the WMS–R (Wechsler, 1988) was consistent with this; her prose recall score on the Logical Memory sub-test was associated with the 5th percentile for immediate recall, and the 3rd percentile for delayed recall. She scored 0/12 on the hard verbal paired associates, and achieved a Verbal MQ of only 69.

One unusual aspect of ROB's memory performance was that her poor verbal recall was not accompanied by a similar deficit on episodic memory tests that required recall of visual or visuo-spatial information. Her Visual MQ was 98, and her performance on the Rey Osterrieth figure was within the normal range. This was very different from the pattern that was observed in Moscovitch's (1989) ACoA patient whose recall impairment was evident in memory for visual as well as verbal material. Dissociations between memory for verbal and visual information are well documented in patients like ROB who have suffered unilateral brain injury (e.g. Milner, 1958, 1967). As Milner (1967) points out, however, patients with material-specific memory disorders following unilateral temporal lobe damage perform badly regardless of whether memory is assessed by tests of recall or recognition.

This made ROB's entirely preserved performance on tests of recognition memory all the more striking. Her scores of 47/50 on the RMT for words and 46/50 on the RMT for faces were both above the mean score of normal controls. On a series of additional recognition memory tests, ROB consistently performed within the normal range regardless of whether the materials comprised words or nonwords. On subsequent tests of free recall, however, ROB was generally unable to recall any words whatsoever whenever a delay of a couple of minutes was employed between recall and testing, and only a very small number of words when the recall test immediately followed presentation of the last list item.

An Encoding Deficit?

It was therefore clear that the case of ROB represented a dissociation between recall and recognition of verbal material that was as striking as any that had previously been reported. One of the first questions that we investigated was whether ROB's poor recall might be associated with the use of inappropriate encoding strategies. We therefore gave her some verbal paired associates to learn and compared her performance before and after she had been given detailed instructions on how to integrate the pairs using interactive imagery techniques. On another occasion, we gave her a list of unrelated words and made her perform encoding strategies of the kind that Craik and Tulving (1975) used to demonstrate levels of processing effects. Finally, we gave her a passage of prose (Goetz, 1979) and asked her to summarise the main points in the form of written notes to ensure adequate comprehension of the passage. The results of these experiments were strikingly similar; ROB continued to recall verbal information at floor level even when she had clearly employed what most memory researchers would consider to be highly effective encoding strategies.

It would have been useful to have been able to investigate in greater detail the nature of ROB's recall deficit. For example, would her poor performance be associated with an inability to use organisational retrieval strategies at the time of recall (cf Stuss, et al., 1994)? Unfortunately, however, ROB's impairment in the recall of verbal material was so severe that floor effects made it very difficult to make comparisons of this kind. For the rest of this paper therefore, we will concentrate on ROB's apparently preserved recognition memory performance.

An Artefact of Test Difficulty?

One of the key issues raised by Aggleton and Shaw (1996) was the extent to which selective recall deficits might reflect a mild version of the amnesic state. Because recognition tests are generally easier than recall tests, it is possible that preserved recognition memory in such patients might be explained in terms of recognition tests being insufficiently sensitive to detect "milder" memory impairments. As Mayes (1988) pointed out, no attempt is typically made to match test difficulty when a patient's performance on the two types of test is being compared.

In order to address this issue with ROB, we employed a procedure that had previously been used by Calev (1984) to equate the difficulty of the recall and recognition tests that he used to assess memory function in patients categorised as suffering from schizophrenia. Calev gave his subjects a recall test in which they had to learn and then free recall a list of 24 words. In order to make the recall test as easy as possible, all the target words came from six semantic categories, which were blocked together at presentation. Subjects were also given a separate list of 40 uncategorised words to learn which they subsequently had to recognise. Calev selected 24 of these 40 words as critical items. His 40 control subjects produced a mean recognition score for these 24 critical items (15.1) that was very similar to the mean number of words that they remembered in the free recall test (15.6).

ROB was therefore asked to learn 40 words as they appeared one at a time on a VDU, and was then given a recognition test in which she was presented with the 40 targets mixed up with 40 distractors one at a time in a random order. Half of the distractors rhymed with one of the targets, and half of the distractors were related in meaning to one of the target words. She was asked to indicate which were the words that she had just been asked to learn in a single item yes/no recognition test. When recognition was complete, ROB was shown a further list containing 24 words of high frequency that she was asked to learn and then free recall. She successfully recognised 16/24 of the critical items on the recognition test, but scored only 8/24 correct on the free recall test. Her recognition performance was therefore very similar to the mean score of 15.6 (sd = 4.2) achieved by Calev's controls. Her recall performance was over two standard deviations below the score of 15.1 (sd = 3.3) achieved by Calev's controls, however. A similar pattern emerged when ROB's performance was compared with that of control subjects who were matched with her for sex, age, and educational background.

Having established that ROB's selective recall impairment was not an artefact of test difficulty, the next question concerned the nature of the information that she uses when she makes her recognition memory decisions.

Processes Involved in Recognition Decisions

The precise nature of the functional processes that are involved in recognition judgements has been debated throughout the twentieth century. Theorists such as Hollingworth (1913) and Tulving (1983) have argued that retrieval processes are as vital for successful recognition as they are for recall. Kintsch (1968), conversely, claimed that recognition depends solely on a judgement of familiarity and that the need to search through memory is precisely what distinguishes recall from recognition; recall = search plus recognition: More recently, however, dual process models of recognition (e.g. Jacoby, 1983; Mandler, 1980) have become increasingly popular. According to Mandler and Jacoby, a subject can respond positively on a recognition memory test if the context in which it was originally encoded can be retrieved from the target item, or if the target word itself feels more familiar to the subject than it would had it not been present on the list.

It would follow from dual process models of recognition that if a patient were to suffer from difficulties in retrieving information from episodic memory, this could lead to a more severe deficit on tests of recall than recognition. A disproportionately strong recall impairment would be observed if the ability to make familiarity decisions was preserved in such a patient. This issue has recently been investigated by Parkin et al. (1994) with patient CB. When CB was given the same version of the Calev test as that used with ROB, he performed much worse than normal controls on both the test of recognition and the test of recall. However, when the nature of the recognition test was changed from a yes–no test to a forced choice test, then the results were very different. CB now showed unimpaired recognition performance even though his recall score was once again outside the normal range.

According to Parkin et al. (1994, p.39), the explanation for this pattern of performance lies in the extent to which the two recognition tests require contextual retrieval. If the target item is presented simultaneously with the distractors (as in a forced choice test), Parkin et al. argue that the *relative* familiarity of targets and distractors can be assessed. Because relative familiarity will be much more difficult to judge on a yes–no test where items are presented singly at recognition, contextual retrieval will assume greater importance than familiarity judgements. Consequently, Parkin et al. argue that CB is impaired at the use of contextual retrieval during recognition but retains the ability to make familiarity decisions. This leads to problems on yes–no recognition tests, but normal performance on forced-choice tests.

In light of these findings, we thought that it would be interesting to investigate in more detail ROB's performance on different types of recognition memory test. The critical questions were whether she, like CB, would show evidence of significantly better performance on forced choice than yes–no recognition tests (Experiment 1), and whether her recognition might show evidence of disproportionately strong reliance on familiarity judgements rather than contextual retrieval (Experiment 2).

EXPERIMENT 1:
FORCED CHOICE VS YES–NO RECOGNITION TESTS

Method

ROB learnt four different lists of words on four different testing sessions, each one separated by at least two weeks. All of the lists contained 20 words that were presented one at a time on cards for three seconds. The instructions informed her that this was a test of memory and that she should read each word aloud as it was presented and try to remember it. Testing took place one hour after list presentation.

For two of the lists, a forced choice recognition memory test was then administered; ROB was presented with 20 cards one at a time, on each of which was written one of the target words together with two distractors. Order of targets and distractors was counterbalanced. The instructions told her to indicate which of the three words she had read aloud and tried to remember an hour earlier. If necessary, she was asked to guess.

For two of the lists, a yes–no recognition test was administered; ROB was presented with 60 cards one at a time, on each of which was written one word: 20 of the cards contained a target word and 40 contained distractor items. ROB was told to respond "yes" if the word was one of those that she had read aloud and tried to remember an hour earlier, and "no" if it was not. "Don't know" responses were not permitted.

The distractors from all four of the recognition tests comprised 20 items that were related to the target items and 20 unrelated items. For two of the tests (one forced choice, and one yes–no), these were items that rhymed with the targets (e.g. *liner: minor*), and for two of the tests (one forced choice, and one yes–no), these were items that were semantically related to the targets (e.g. *link: connect*). The materials for this test were kindly loaned to us by Alan Parkin and Claire Bindschaedler.

Results and Discussion

The results of this experiment are summarised in Table 6.1. It can be seen that the level of performance achieved by ROB is strikingly similar regardless of the type of recognition test that was used. On both forced choice and yes–no tests, she correctly recognised .70 of the target items overall. The number of distractor items that she falsely recognised was also very similar, .30 on the forced choice tests, and .35 on the yes–no tests.

These results therefore provide no evidence that ROB has any greater impairment on yes–no tests than on forced choice tests. The results of this experiment therefore suggest that the differences between ROB (Hanley et al., 1994) and CB (Parkin et al., 1994) that were observed on the standard version of the Calev test can also be observed on other tests of recognition memory. CB performs much better on forced choice tests than on yes–no tests; for ROB, however, the nature of the recognition memory test does not seem to be important.

According to Parkin et al. (1994), CB's superior performance on forced choice tests suggests a particular deficit in the contextual retrieval component of recognition memory. This is because Parkin et al. assume that familiarity decisions can be used to perform forced choice tests successfully, but that yes–no decisions require contextual recognition because targets and distractors are not presented to subjects simultaneously. It follows from this account that ROB's ability to perform contextual retrieval when making recognition memory decisions is relatively unimpaired.

If this is true, then it would be expected that ROB's recognition performance would not show evidence of disproportionate reliance on the use of familiarity decisions. An alternative possibility is that CB has a mild deficit in the use of familiarity decisions that impairs performance on yes–no tasks, but not on forced choice tests. If this were to be the case then it remains possible that neither CB nor ROB can use contextual retrieval, and that ROB's

TABLE 6.1
The number of words that ROB successfully recognised in
Experiment 1 in forced choice and yes–no recognition tests.

	Forced choice test		Yes–No test	
	Hits	False Alarms	Hits	False Alarms
Semantic Distractors	.65	.35	.80	.30
Rhyme Distractors	.75	.25	.60	.35
Overall	.70	.30	.70	.33

superior performance on yes–no tests reflects a more fully preserved ability to make familiarity decisions. In Experiment 2 this issue was investigated by the use of Gardiner's *remember/know* paradigm.

EXPERIMENT 2 :
THE REMEMBER/KNOW DISTINCTION

Gardiner (1988) asked subjects to provide information about the nature of their recollective experience when they were performing recognition decisions. He asked them to distinguish between "remember" responses and "know" responses. A "remember" response was used by subjects to indicate a positive recognition decision that was based on specific recollection of some aspect of what happened when the target item was originally presented. A "know" response indicated a positive recognition decision that occurred in the absence of any specific recollective experience of what happened at encoding.

Gardiner (1988) established the validity of this procedure by demonstrating that certain variables increased the number of "remember" responses made by subjects without affecting the number of "know" responses that they made. Of particular importance is the finding (e.g. Parkin & Walter, 1992; Perfect, Williams, & Anderton-Brown, 1995) that elderly subjects typically make a greater number of "know" decisions, and fewer "remember" decisions than younger subjects, even when overall level of recognition is similar in the two subject groups. This is consistent with the view that older subjects are more likely to use recognition decisions based on familiarity, whereas younger subjects are more likely to use contextual retrieval.

In Experiment 2, we used the distinction between "know" and "remember" responses to investigate the nature of the recognition memory decisions that ROB makes. If she performs in a similar way to elderly subjects and makes a relatively large number of "know" responses, this would suggest that her recognition memory relies disproportionately on familiarity decisions. On the basis of her performance in Experiment 1, however, it was predicted that she should show normal levels of "remember" and "know" responses.

Method

The procedure used was identical to that employed by Gardiner and Parkin (1990). ROB was presented with 36 words one at a time, on cards, at a rate of one word every two seconds. As they were presented, ROB was told to "attend to the words and try to remember them". There then followed a 10-minute retention interval, during which time ROB and the experimenter engaged in conversation.

At the end of the retention interval, ROB was given a sheet of paper that contained the 36 target words mixed in with 36 distractors. She was told to work through the list, picking the words that she recognised from the pack she had been shown earlier. For each item she recognised, ROB was asked to indicate whether the decision was based on remembering some thought about the word that she had had when it was shown on the card during learning, or whether she simply knew that the word was part of the list without remembering any thought about the word at encoding. In the former situation she was told to write "R", and in the latter situation to write "K" next to the appropriate word. The *remember/know* instructions followed exactly those used by Gardiner and Parkin (1990). ROB showed every sign of understanding fully the nature of these instructions. The materials used in this experiment were kindly loaned to us by Alan Parkin.

Results and Discussion

The performance of ROB in this experiment together with the mean scores achieved by Gardiner and Parkin's (1990) normal subjects are summarised in Table 6.2. It can be seen that ROB's overall level of recognition is towards the bottom of the normal range. The pattern of performance that she shows is dramatically different from that of Gardiner and Parkin's (1990) normal subjects, however. ROB made no "remember" responses whatsoever; all of her recognition decisions consisted of "know" responses. These results suggest that ROB's recognition memory decisions are dependent on familiarity decisions rather than on contextual retrieval. They are therefore consistent with the view that her selective recall impairment reflects a difficulty in contextual recollection despite a normal ability to make familiarity decisions. Nevertheless, this result ran counter to our predictions, and appears difficult to reconcile with the findings of Experiment 1. Might there be some alternative reason why ROB made no "remember" responses in this experiment?

TABLE 6.2
The number of *remember* and *know* decisions made by ROB in Experiment 2 using Gardiner and Parkin's (1990) procedure (max = 36).

	Hits		False Alarms	
	Remember	Know	Remember	Know
ROB	0	28	0	5
Controls	25.70	5.65	0.25	1.65
SD	4.50	3.26	0.44	1.87

Perfect et al. (1995) have argued that the reason why elderly subjects make fewer "remember" and more "know" decisions is that they are more likely than younger subjects to engage in shallow encoding strategies such as rote rehearsal when they are attempting to learn the words. When they used an orienting task to ensure that older subjects would encode the words semantically, Perfect et al. showed that the older subjects made a similar proportion of "know" and "remember" responses to the young subjects. It is therefore possible that ROB's pattern of performance on this test reflects the use of low-level encoding strategies during learning rather than an inability to use contextual retrieval during recognition. Consistently with this, ROB did inform the experimenters at the end of the recognition test that she had simply repeated the words to herself at encoding, and had made no "remember" decisions because she had not had any unique thoughts about any of the words during learning.

This raises the question of whether the number of "remember" responses that ROB makes would be increased if she performed a semantic orienting task on the words at encoding. It is therefore interesting to report the results of a further experiment that we have conducted with ROB using the know/ remember distinction. In this experiment, the Warrington (1984) recognition memory test for words was again administered to ROB, but this time ROB was asked to indicate whether she was making her recognition decisions on the basis of a "remember" or a "know" decision. The use of the Warrington test is particularly interesting in the light of this discussion because in it the subject is asked to make "pleasantness" judgements about each of the target words at encoding. This ensures that the words are being processed semantically. Under these conditions, ROB correctly recognised 49/50 of the words, making 47 "remember" decisions and 2 "know" decisions.

The results of these two tests have therefore yielded strikingly different results. On the Warrington test, ROB made virtually no "know" responses. When the Gardiner and Parkin (1990) procedure was used, she made no "remember" responses whatsoever. There would appear to be three possible explanations for such a pattern of performance. The first is that ROB was confused by the nature of the distinction that she was being asked to make, and interpreted the instructions differently on the two testing occasions. Although we cannot rule out this possibility, our impression at the times of testing was that ROB understood the instructions perfectly well.

The second possibility is that the different ratio of "know" and "remember" responses came about because of the use of a yes–no recognition test in the Gardiner and Parkin procedure, and a forced choice test in the Warrington procedure. It is unfortunate that the two tests differed in this way, particularly as the literature does not contain any systematic attempts to investigate the effects of different types of recognition test on the incidence of "remember" and "know" decisions. However, there appear to be little grounds for believing that forced choice tests might make a subject more likely to use a "remember" response. If anything, one might have expected that the opposite would be the case (cf. Parkin et al., 1994).

We therefore believe that it is most likely that it was the use of a semantic orienting task that increased the number of "remember" responses that ROB made when the Warrington procedure was employed. In this respect, we would argue that ROB's performance is consistent with that which Perfect et al. (1995) observed in their elderly subjects, although ROB showed an even more dramatic shift towards "know" responses when the Gardiner and Parkin (1990) procedure was used than is observed in elderly subjects (Parkin & Walter, 1992; Perfect et al., 1995).

ROB's consistent use of "remember" rather than "know" responses when performing the Warrington recognition memory test suggests that she is able to use contextual retrieval as the basis for recognition memory decisions. This conclusion is consistent with the view that preserved recognition in ROB has a quite different basis from preserved recognition in CB (Parkin et al., 1994). Although it would clearly be interesting to examine ROB's use of "remember" and "know" judgements in further experiments, we believe the evidence favours the view that her recognition memory skills are essentially unimpaired. It seems to be the case that ROB can use both familiarity and contextual retrieval as the basis for recognition memory decisions, whereas CB appears to rely much more heavily on familiarity decisions.

CONCLUSION

An important question about patients such as ROB is whether they are best considered as suffering from a form of the amnesic syndrome. Previously we have argued that there are a number of reasons why this does not seem appropriate (Hanley et al., 1994; Hanley & Young, 1994). For example, the areas of the brain to which ACoA patients such as ROB and CB have suffered injury are different from those that are associated with the amnesic syndrome (Parkin & Leng, 1993; Parkin et al., 1994). These patients appear to have lesions to the frontal cortex or the basal ganglia rather than injuries to the midline regions that are associated with amnesia. In common with Parkin and his colleagues (Parkin et al., 1993; Parkin et al., 1994), we previously argued that the account that best fits ROB's pattern of performance is provided by Shallice (1988). In Shallice's terms, ROB can be seen as suffering from an impairment at the level of the supervisory system.

Shallice (1988 p.378) argues that a supervisory system located in the frontal lobes plays a key role in enabling the episodic store to function effectively. The supervisory system is considered to be responsible for setting up detailed retrieval strategies that enable desired information to be accessed in episodic memory. In addition, the supervisory system also has a critical role in determining whether or not information that is retrieved from episodic memory is appropriate. Patients with impairments to this system will therefore suffer from problems that are "concerned with formulating the description of any memories that might be required, and of verifying that any candidate memories that are retrieved are relevant".

If Shallice is correct, then it would follow that there are two ways in which a supervisory system breakdown could impair memory performance. First, it might lead to a problem with the use of retrieval strategies that would allow access to information stored in episodic memory on tasks such as free recall. This is the pattern of impairment observed in ROB. Second, a supervisory system breakdown could lead to a difficulty in the accurate evaluation of information that is retrieved from episodic store. This would not necessarily reduce recall, but would be likely to result in recognition memory problems, and the tendency for a subject to confabulate. This is precisely the pattern of impairment that was observed by Delbecq-Derouesné, Beauvois, and Shallice (1990) in another patient (RW) who had also suffered a left hemisphere ACoA. RW experienced exactly the opposite memory impairment from that observed in ROB; his recall performance was normal apart from a tendency to include a large number of intrusions. His performance on tests of recognition memory, including that of Warrington (1984), was severely impaired, however. The existence of this double dissociation between RW and ROB provides strong evidence for Shallice's conceptualisation of the role of the supervisory system in memory function.

Recently an alternative characterisation of memory impairments that are associated with damage to frontal lobe structures has been proposed by Norman and Schacter (1996). Norman and Schacter agree that the frontal system plays a key role in memory retrieval and in monitoring information that has been retrieved from memory. However, they do not believe that the processes involved in retrieval and in monitoring should be as sharply distinguished as they were by Delbecq-Derouesné et al. (1990), Hanley et al. (1994), and Shallice (1988). This is because both retrieval and monitoring "depend on reinstating (in a top-down fashion) contextual information associated with the target episode" (1996, p.240). That is, in a task that depends on retrieval such as free recall, the subject must generate contextual constraints that can be used as retrieval cues for the to-be-remembered material. In a task (e.g. recognition) that depends on monitoring, the subject must generate contextual information from the target item in order to determine that it is an "old" item rather than a distractor. Such similarities suggest to Norman and Schacter (1996, p.241) that it "may not be necessary to assign strategic retrieval and monitoring to separate neural circuits".

Such an account can provide a clear explanation of the performance of patient CB (Parkin et al., 1994), who fares badly on tests of recall and on yes–no recognition tests, but performs relatively well on forced choice recognition tests. According to Norman and Schacter, CB has a general problem in the generation of context but performs well on forced choice tests because these can be accomplished on the basis of familiarity decisions.

In contrast to patients such as CB who suffer from a total failure to retrieve context, Norman and Schacter argue that there are patients who suffer from a partial failure to retrieve contextual constraints. They claim that patient BG (Schacter et al., 1996) who makes an excessive number of false alarms on tests of recognition memory is only able to generate extremely vague contextual constraints. They argue that limited contextual knowledge (e.g. information about the semantic categories from which the target words were drawn) prevents him from making false alarms to distractors from non-studied categories, but makes him vulnerable to non-studied items from studied categories.

Norman and Schacter offer no specific explanation of the type of memory impairment that is observed in patient ROB, however. ROB's unimpaired performance on yes–no recognition tests such as the Calev test suggests that her ability to generate context in recognition is normal despite her extremely poor free recall performance. Why should top-down generation of context be impaired in free recall but not in recognition if the same frontal system subserves performance on both tasks? Norman and Schacter make an important point that we entirely accept when they argue that both retrieval and monitoring involve top-down generation of contextual constraints. However, the way in which context is generated in free recall and in recognition may make very different types of demands on the frontal memory system. Although it may be less parsimonious, we believe that the empirical evidence as it currently stands favours the view that functionally distinct components of the frontal memory system subserve performance on recall and on yes–no recognition tasks.

The preceding discussion suggests some potentially fruitful ideas for future experimental work with patients such as ROB. We have argued that ROB's preserved recognition on yes–no tests occurs because it requires a form of contextual retrieval that is different from that which is involved in free recall. In certain types of memory paradigm, however, the retrieval demands of the recall and recognition tests are much more similar than they are in the experiments reported in this paper and by Hanley et al. (1994). Consequently, it would be interesting to observe ROB's recognition performance in tests of the kind that were used by Tulving and his colleagues to demonstrate recognition failure of recallable words (see Tulving, 1983). In these experiments, each target word is encoded in the context of a unique cue word and recognition of the target word takes place in the absence of the cue words. The contextual retrieval operations that are involved in a recognition test such as this appear to be very similar to those that are involved in cued recall. If our account is correct, then a recognition test of this kind may pose severe problems for ROB.

Norman and Schacter offer some additional ideas concerning modality-specific memory deficits in patients with frontal lobe or basal ganglia damage. Here, we are in close agreement with their suggestions. It was stated earlier that ROB's recall problems were specific to verbal material. In the terminology of Shallice (1988), it might be considered counterintuitive that a supervisory system impairment could prevent recall of verbal but not visual material. Norman and Schacter argue that the nature of the information (e.g. visual features) that might be used to provide the contextual constraints that would enable recall of pictorial material are likely to be radically different from those that would be used to recall verbal material. In these terms, modality-specific retrieval impairments in patients with unilateral injuries to the frontal cortex or basal ganglia are exactly what would be predicted (see also Milner, Corsi, & Leonard, 1991).

In summary, our main claim is that anterograde amnesia is best seen as being the result of a failure to register new information in episodic memory (e.g. Tulving & Schacter, 1990) as a result of brain injuries associated with the diencephalic midline. Investigations of patients such as CB, RW, and ROB, however, have revealed no evidence of injury in this region of the brain. Moreover, the memory performance of such patients can be comfortably within the normal range on standard tests of episodic memory function, even when steps are taken to ensure that such tests are as difficult as those on which they perform badly. This appears to rule out the possibility that their impairments reflect a failure to store information in episodic memory. Instead, we believe that their problems stem from an inability to make appropriate use of stored information whenever the memory test requires the use of subject-initiated retrieval strategies to access episodic memory (e.g. ROB) or the specific requirement to monitor what has been retrieved (RW) from episodic memory. The question of whether monitoring and retrieval reflect the operation of functionally separate components of the frontal memory system is an important issue for future research to address.

REFERENCES

Aggleton, J.P., & Shaw, C. (1996). Amnesia and recognition memory: A re-analysis of psychometric data. *Neuropsychologia, 34,* 51–62.

Calev, A., (1984). Recall and recognition in chronic nondemented schizophrenics. *Journal of Abnormal Psychology, 93,* 172–177.

Craik, F.I.M., & Tulving, E. (1975). Depth of processing and the retention of words in episodic memory. *Journal of Experimental Psychology: General, 104,* 268–294.

Delbecq-Derouesné, J., Beauvois, M.F. & Shallice, T. (1990). Preserved recall versus impaired recognition. *Brain, 13*, 1045–1074.

DeLuca, J., & Cicerone, K.D. (1991). Confabulation following aneurysm of the anterior communicating artery. *Cortex, 27*, 417–423.

Gardiner, J.M. (1988). Functional aspects of recollective experience. *Memory & Cognition, 16*, 309–313.

Gardiner, J.M., & Parkin, A.J. (1990). Attention and recollective experience in recognition memory. *Memory & Cognition, 18*, 579–583.

Goetz, E.T. (1979). Inferring from text: Some factors influencing which inferences will be made. *Discourse Processes, 2*, 179–195.

Hanley, J.R., Davies, A.D.M., Downes, J., & Mayes, A. (1994). Impaired recall of verbal material following an anterior communicating artery aneurysm. *Cognitive Neuropsychology, 11*, 543–578.

Hanley, J.R., & Young, A.W. (1994). The cognitive neuropsychology of memory. In P.E. Morris & M. Gruneberg (Eds.), *Theoretical aspects of memory* (2nd Edn.) London: Routledge.

Hollingworth, H.L. (1913). Characteristic differences between recall and recognition. *American Journal of Psychology, 24*, 532–544.

Jacoby, L.L. (1983). Perceptual enhancement: Persistent effects of an experience. *Journal of Experimental Psychology: Learning, Memory and Cognition, 9*, 21–38.

Kintsch, W. (1968). Recognition and free recall of organised lists. *Journal of Experimental Psychology, 78*, 481–487.

Mandler, G. (1980). Recognising: The judgement of previous occurrence. *Psychological Review, 87*, 252–271.

Mayes, A.R. (1988). *Human organic memory disorders.* Cambridge: Cambridge University Press.

Milner, B. (1958). Psychological defects produced by temporal lobe excision. *Research Publications: Association for Research in Nervous and Mental Disease, 36*, 244–257.

Milner, B. (1967). Brain mechanisms suggested by studies of temporal lobes. In C.H. Millikan & F.L. Darley (Eds.), *Brain mechanisms underlying speech and language.* New York & London: Grune & Stratton.

Milner, B., Corsi, P., & Leonard, G. (1991). Frontal-lobe contributions to recency judgements. *Neuropsychologia, 29*, 601–618.

Moscovitch, M. (1989). Confabulation and the frontal systems: Strategic versus associative retrieval in neuropsychological theories of memory. In H.L. Roediger III & F.I.M. Craik (Eds.), *Varieties of memory and consciousness: Essays in honor of Endel Tulving.* Hillsdale, NJ: Lawrence Erlbaum Associates Inc.

Nelson, H. (1982). *The new adult reading test.* Windsor, UK: NFER Publishing Company.

Norman, K.A., & Schacter, D.L. (1996). Implicit memory, explicit memory and false recognition: A cognitive neuroscience perspective. In L.M. Reder (Ed.), *Implicit memory and metacognition.* Hillsdale, NJ: Lawrence Erlbaum Associates Inc.

Parkin, A.J., Dunn, J.C., Lee, C., O'Hara, P.F., & Nussbaum, L. (1993). Neuropsychological sequelae of Wernicke's encephalopathy in a 20-year-old woman: Selective impairment of a frontal memory system. *Brain & Cognition, 21*, 1–19.

Parkin, A.J., & Leng, N.R.C. (1993). *Neuropsychology of the amnesic syndrome.* Hove, UK: Lawrence Erlbaum Associates Ltd.

Parkin, A.J., & Walter, B.M. (1992). Recollective experience, normal ageing and frontal dysfunction. *Psychology & Ageing, 7*, 290–298.

Parkin, A.J., Yeomans, J., & Bindschaedler, C. (1994). Further characterisation of the executive memory impairment following frontal lobe lesions. *Brain & Cognition, 26*, 23–42.

Perfect, T.J., Williams, R.B., & Anderton-Brown, C. (1995). Age differences in reported recollective experience are due to encoding effects, not response bias. *Memory*, *3*, 169–186.

Robinson, J.A. (1976). Sampling autobiographical memory. *Cognitive Psychology*, *8*, 578–595.

Schacter, D.L., Curran, T., Galluccio, L Milberg, W.P., & Bates, J. (1996). False recognition and the right frontal lobe: A case study. *Neuropsychologia*, *34*, 793–808.

Shallice, T. (1988). *From neuropsychology to mental structure.* Cambridge: Cambridge University Press.

Stuss, D.T., Alexander, M.P., Palumbo, C.P., Buckle, L., Sayer, L., & Pogue, J. (1994). Organisational strategies of patients with unilateral or bilateral frontal lobe injury in word list learning tasks. *Neuropsychology*, *8*, 355–373.

Tulving, E. (1983). *Elements of episodic memory.* New York: Oxford University Press.

Tulving, E. & Schacter, D.L. (1990). Priming and human memory systems. *Science*, *247*, 301–306.

Warrington, E.K. (1984). *Recognition memory test.* Windsor, UK: NFER-Nelson.

Warrington, E.K. & Weislantz, L. (1970). The amnesic syndrome: Consolidation or retrieval? *Nature*, *228*, 628–630.

Wechsler, D. (1981). *Wechsler Adult Intelligence Scale–Revised.* New York: Psychological Corp.

Wechsler, D. (1988). *Wechsler Memory Scale–Revised.* New York: Harcourt Brace Jovanovitch.

7 The Long and Winding Road: Twelve Years of Frontal Amnesia

Alan J. Parkin
University of Sussex, UK

INTRODUCTION

If asked to name a famous brain-damaged patient, most psychologists would think of Phineas Gage whose unfortunate accident in 1848 has a special place in the annals of science. For those of you who do not know the story, Gage was a railroad engineer whose job involved laying and detonating explosive. This process involved use of a tamping iron to pack explosive into a bore hole. One day, while using the iron, the explosive detonated and sent the iron bar straight through Gage's head, resulting in extensive damage to his frontal lobes. What surprised everybody was the outcome—at a time when medicine was so primitive one would not expect anyone to survive such a terrible injury[1] but, "he was alive at two o'clock the next afternoon, in full possession of his reason, and free from pain."

However, as all students know, all was not well with Phineas Gage: his personality had changed. Harlow (1868/1993, p.227) the physician who attended Gage, noted that "his equilibrium, or balance, so to speak, between his intellectual faculties and animal propensities seems to have been destroyed. He is fitful, irreverent, indulging in the grossest profanity (which was not previously his custom), manifesting but little deference for his fellows, impatient of restraint or advice when it conflicts with his desires." In short he was "no longer Gage". Gage's impromptu psychosurgery had clearly

[1]It is now thought that Gage survived because the heat of the tamping iron cauterised the wound, thus freeing it from infection.

127

changed his personality and this led to the idea that the social behaviour of humans could be altered by operating on the human brain. In 1890 the surgeon Burckhart was the first to believe that removing parts of the frontal lobe could alleviate psychiatric symptoms and this tradition culminated in the widespread use of frontal leucotomy during the 1930s and 1940s.

There can be no doubt that the reckless procedures carried out on the frontal lobes by neurosurgeons would have been modified if they had realised that the frontal lobes were implicated in more essential functions. Yet, even if they had only looked at accounts of Gage himself they would have spotted something crucial. Commenting on Gage's memory Harlow (p.227) notes that Gage "was accustomed to entertain his little nephews and nieces with the most fabulous recitals of wonderful feats and hair breadth escapes, without any foundation except in his fancy". From our modern perspective we can identify these fabrications as a memory disorder known as confabulation—one of the memory problems associated with damage to the frontal lobes.

Sadly that single sentence is the only known comment on Gage's memory, so our ideas about how his memory might have been impaired can only come from studying patients who have suffered damage similar to that inflicted by the famous tamping iron. I have been fortunate to work with such a case, JB, and in addition, I have been able to follow him for the last 12 years, thus allowing me to observe how his memory problems have changed and how they have affected his life.

CASE JB

JB was born in 1943 and had a conventional grammar school education followed by a range of jobs mainly in the entertainment industry. At the age of 42 he suffered a ruptured ACoA aneurysm. Following its repair a large left frontal horn with an adjacent low-density area was detected by CAT scan. Unfortunately the extent of aneurysmal clipping (three clips used) prevented detailed neuroradiological assessment, but minimally, JB was considered to have damage to the left frontal cortex and the left caudate nucleus (Parkin, Leng, Stanhope, & Smith, 1988).

My first encounter with JB was extremely memorable. Like so many acutely confused patients he had been hospitalised and had been sedated with major tranquillisers. I recall giving him the Anna Thompson story to recall. He very quickly went off the point and started to confabulate. When I told him the session was over he said he knew the way back and promptly walked into a broom cupboard. At that stage his confusion was such that he believed himself to be in his 20s and, for example, that he was planning to get married. In fact he had been divorced many years previously. Over and over again his behaviour was guided by the belief that he was in his 20s. His father had died some years previously yet he would insist that he had just had a drink with him that lunchtime. When told his father was dead he would shrug his shoulders nonchalantly and remark that there was someone down the pub who looked just like his father.

A feature of JB's confabulation was that he tended to superimpose his more stable past on to his present, thus creating bizarre blended memories in which, for example, the hospital he was in became a college:

AP: Tell me a bit about [name of hospital].
JB: Well it's a nuthouse for want of a better phrase—lunatic asylum I would imagine.
AP: What makes you say that?
JB: There's some funny people in there. I want out.
AP: You were telling me about [name of hospital]. Why do you think you're there?
JB: I don't really know. I have asked several people but never got an answer that satisfies me. Don't know why I'm there at all.
AP: What do you do during the day there?
JB: Same as everyone else. Bit of maths, bit of English, bit of religion first thing in the morning ... depends what's on the timetable—normal school lessons.
AP: If it's a nuthouse why are you having lessons?
JB: Brain stimulation I suppose.
AP: Brain stimulation?
JB: Got to get the brain working again.

JB's variable insight interacting with confabulation also cropped up a little later in the same conversation:

JB: I've been chugging along over the last three weeks ... It's this bloody memory.
AP: Memory's the problem?
JB: Yea.
AP: You're confused about where you are. You would like some help?
JB: Yea, clear the old brain from where it's got clogged up.
AP: How often do you find yourself confused?
JB: Quite regularly. Sort of get in the car and think where am I going? I must sit and work it all out. But it's not as bad as all that—I'll retract that straight away.
AP: What helps then?
JB: Well I give myself a clue and I can work it out from there. Well I've got in the car and looked at my timetable where it says on the first page which school I'm going to. I haven't turned up at the wrong one yet.
AP: How many different schools do you go to?
JB: Well there's been three in as many months.

By 1987 JB's confused confabulatory state had ameliorated and left him with a milder range of cognitive impairments, which have remained largely unchanged ever since. JB's continuing memory impairment has resulted in an extreme tendency for him to repeat himself and this makes it very difficult to spend any amount of time with him. It is not unusual for him to tell an elaborate anecdote and then, within a matter of minutes, embark on the same anecdote without any apparent sense of it being familiar. Despite JB's good performance on frontal lobe tests (see later) even 10 minutes of conversation is sufficient to confirm his frontal pathology because he exhibits markedly disinhibited behaviour. Thus he will talk to anyone regardless of what they think of him and can often make socially unacceptable statements. As a result he has been excluded from all the local public houses but, through an enduring lack of insight, fails to understand why. When asked to explain why he does not work he usually relies on cliches such as "My get up and go has got up and gone"—only rarely will he mention that he had an aneurysm but he has little ability to explain the implication of this. He also shows a classic lack of planning ability. As far as cooking goes he can do little more than boil an egg and his financial matters are handled by a solicitor. What money he has he spends almost immediately—most of it on lottery tickets and slot machines. We have tried to get him to buy food but he spends many days without eating much at all. His appearance is dishevelled but this does not seem to worry him. He often fails to respond appropriately when some form of emotional response is needed. For example, when I told him that my father had just died he greeted this news with complete indifference. JB's impairments have precluded any gainful employment and he spends his days walking around his home town following a set route. We estimate that he walks about 12 miles every day.

Table 7.1 shows JB's performance on the Wechsler Adult Intelligence Scale–Revised (WAIS–R; Wechsler, 1981) and it can be seen that there has been no significant decline in intelligence relative to his estimated pre-morbid IQ (NART; Nelson, 1985). He also performs extremely well on the Standard Progressive Matrices (Raven, 1960). On the Wechsler Memory Scale–Revised (WMS–R; Wechsler, 1984) JB shows marked impairments on both tests of logical memory, paired associates, and the delayed visual reproduction test. Examination of Table 7.1 shows that JB's indices are comparable to patients with Wernicke–Korsakoff Syndrome in verbal memory, general memory, and delayed recall.

Additional testing confirmed findings from WMS–R that JB's deficit is worse for verbal than non-verbal material. On the Warrington Recognition Memory Test (Warrington, 1984) he scored 30/50 for words (percentile < 5) but on faces he scored 39/50 (percentile 10). On the Rey Auditory Verbal Learning Test (Rey, 1964) he achieved 23 correct across five immediate

TABLE 7.1
IB's Profile on WAIS–R and WMS–R

WAIS–R			
Verbal		*Performance*	
Information	10	Picture completion	9
Digit span	10	Picture arrangement	8
Vocabulary	12	Block design	11
Arithmetic	15	Object assembly	10
Comprehension	11	Digit symbol	9
Similarities	12		
Verbal IQ	113	Performance IQ	107
Full scale IQ	110		
National Adult Reading Test estimated pre-morbid IQ 117			

WMS–R				
Percentiles		*Indices*		
Digits Forward	28	Verbal Memory	68	(70)
Digits Backward	29	Visual Memory	88	(77)
Visual Span Forward	99	General Memory	68	(68)
Visual Span Backward	71	Delayed Recall	55	(57)
Logical Memory	9	Attention/Concentration	105	(91)
Logical Memory Delay	<1			
Visual Reproduction	54			
Visual Reproduction Delay	5			

Figures in parentheses indicate mean performance of eight Korsakoff patients (Wechsler, 1984).

recall trials with 14 intrusions and a delayed recall of two items and four intrusions. On the Rey Figure copying was slightly abnormal (see Parkin & Leng, 1993, p.22) but immediate retention was between percentile 10 and 30 dropping to percentile 3.5 after 30 minutes.

On tests of frontal function JB was found to be normal on the modified Wisconsin Card Sorting Test (Nelson, 1976), 6 categories, 0 perseverative errors; normal on FAS word fluency (Benton & Hamsher, 1976), 52. He was unimpaired on cognitive estimation (Shallice & Evans, 1978), 3; normal on the Stroop Test (Trenerry, Crosson, DeBoe, & Leber, 1989), percentile 78; and within normal limits on the Ruff figural fluency test (Ruff, Light, & Evans, 1987), 45 correct reproductions and no perseveration. However, JB did exhibit problems with the Alternative Uses Test (Guildford, Christensen, Merrifield, & Wilson, 1978) in which he produced only six acceptable uses, although this is significantly above the score of 1.5 reported in Eslinger and Grattan's (1993) frontal lobe group.

INVESTIGATIONS OF JB

For the last nine years we have been looking at JB's memory to try and understand why it is so poor. Table 7.1 shows that many of JB's memory scores are similar to patients with Wernicke–Korsakoff Syndrome, but to describe JB as having an amnesic syndrome would be very misleading. JB does remember quite a lot including, for example, various cars I have owned over the years. He also remembers and can describe the various colleagues who have accompanied me and tested him. None of this would be expected from a patient with an amnesic syndrome.

The key to understanding JB's impairment came from an observation made by my colleague Claire Bindschaedler who had been studying how he performed on a variety of recognition tests. She noticed that he tended to show a normal or slightly above average hit rate but that his false alarm rate was around 40% (see Table 7.2). This was unusual and, at that time, had not been documented elsewhere. We set out to try and understand why this was occurring.

One of our first experiments involved a pair of tests designed by Claudia Metzler and stimuli from these are illustrated in Fig. 7.1. In the non-distracting (ND) condition, targets and distractors are designed so that they share no overlapping features. In the distracting (D) condition, each target has a corresponding distractor which differs from its target by only one feature. At test a random sequence comprising targets and distractors is presented individually and the subject is required to indicate whether or not each item is a target. JB's results on this task were very striking. On the ND condition his hit rate was 77% (control 96%) with no false alarms; however, on the D condition he made 61% hits (80%) but with a false alarm rate of 67% (36%) (see Parkin, Bindschaedler, Harsent, & Metzler, 1996).

This result was interesting because it indicated that JB's high false alarm rate was not just a wilful tendency to say "yes" regardless of circumstances. Instead it suggested that this high false alarm rate was determined by the relationship between targets and distractors. When there was overlap in content he made high false alarms, when there was no overlap he was able to perform within normal limits.

TABLE 7.2
Performance by JB on 10 Different
Tests of Yes/No Recognition
(Proportional Data)

	Hits	False Alarms
	.84	.43
SD	.10	.16

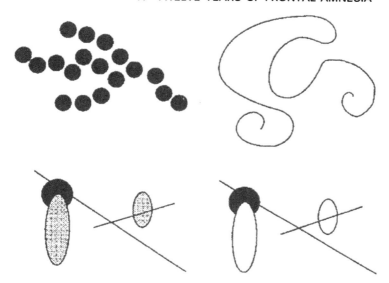

FIG. 7.1. Stimuli from the nondistracting and distracting abstract designs test.

Our initial interpretation of this was that JB's recognition memory must be operating on the basis of familiarity cues. Briefly, it is now widely accepted that recognition is a dual component process involving familiarity information, i.e. information that registers a stimulus as previously encountered, and recollection, in which a familiar stimulus is placed in a specific context. In the ND condition, only the targets have familiar features thus enabling them to be distinguished from distractors solely on the basis of familiarity. In the D condition, however, the high degree of target–distractor overlap would render familiarity obsolete as a cue. It is under these conditions that JB's memory produces abnormal false alarms and thus suggests that he is over-reliant on familiarity.

The distinction between familiarity and recollection has been operationalised in a number of ways. Tulving (1985), for example, required subjects to classify recognised stimuli into two categories "remember" (R) and "know" (K), which, respectively, corresponded to subjective judgements of recollection and familiarity. Subsequent experiments by Gardiner and his colleagues (e.g. Gardiner & Java, 1992) have shown that these subjective distinctions appear to map reliably on to different forms of remembering.

Given data from the abstract designs tests, we were interested in seeing how JB performed when asked to make R and K judgements about recognised stimuli. In a test involving memory for 36 targets his hit rate was 86% (control 83%). Control subjects classified 64% of hits as R and 36% as K. JB classified all his correct hits as K. Predictably his false alarm rate was high at 55% (control 0.4%) and all these were classified as K.

Although we would maintain that JB has largely preserved intelligence, it might be argued that this massive preponderance of K responses arises because he does not understand the instructions rather than because he just finds everything familiar. We therefore conducted a more objective test of the familiarity hypothesis using a modified forced choice procedure. In the experiment subjects studied an initial word list and were then given a forced choice recognition test in which each target had to be discriminated from an unrelated target. In the second critical trial that followed, a new target list was presented but, on forced choice, subjects had to discriminate the new targets from distractors used as targets on trial 1. Under these conditions all items can be assumed to have high levels of familiarity and correct identification depends on the ability to retrieve the correct context of an item. To ensure that any deficit on trial 2 was not due to proactive interference, two additional trials involving non-repeated items were given.

The results are shown in Fig. 7.2 and indicate that JB's performance on the critical trial was at chance despite normal performance on the third and fourth trials. As trial 2 is the only trial where item familiarity would not suffice as a cue to recognition, these results appeared to confirm the familiarity hypothesis of JB's memory deficit.

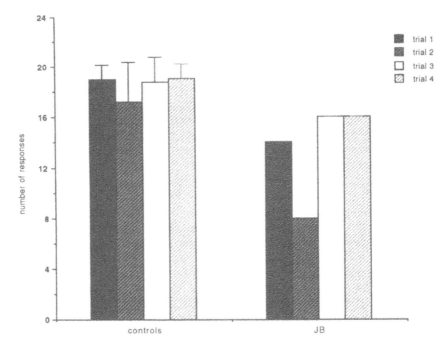

FIG. 7.2. Performance of JB and controls on four successive forced choice trials.

At this point JB's deficit seemed simple enough to explain—he fails to either encode or retrieve contextual information and this makes him over-reliant on familiarity. Straightforward explanations rarely survive in psychology and our investigations of JB are no exception—as became evident when we attempted further tests of the familiarity hypothesis.

Any theory of familiarity-based recognition memory will predict that higher false alarm rates will be encountered on recognition tests which use distractors that have some similarity to targets. Thus if one test contains distractors with similar meaning to targets one would expect higher levels of false alarms compared with the non-overlapping condition. We confidently expected to see this effect in JB by comparing his false alarm rate in a test where distractors were either strong synonyms of targets (e.g. purchase–buy), weak synonyms (e.g. novel–book), or where no overlap was found. The results are shown in Fig 7.3. First note that the manipulation was effective for controls but, for JB, there were as many false alarms in the non-overlapping condition as in the high overlap condition.

A possible explanation of the synonym study was that JB is heavily influenced by previous experiments and, conceivably, some of his false alarms arise because distractors have been used in previous experiments. To get

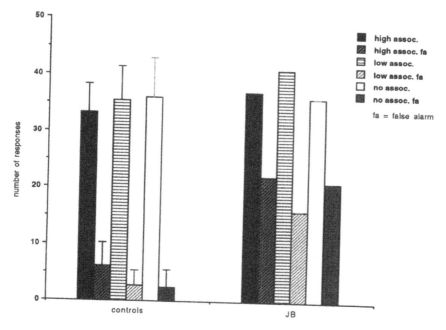

FIG. 7.3. JB's performance compared with controls on the synonym distractor task.

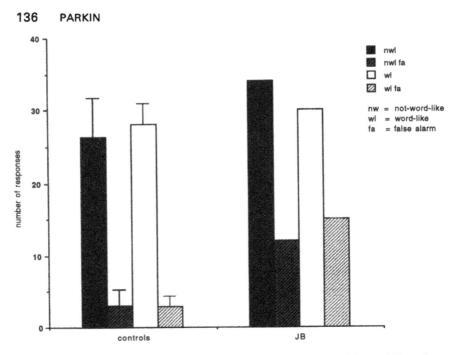

FIG. 7.4. JB's performance compared with controls on a recognition test involving word-like and not-word-like nonwords.

around this problem we conducted a second experiment in which JB studied nonwords. Two types of nonword were used. Those that looked like real words (e.g. pronce) and those that did not (e.g. tunjate). Figure 7.4 shows that his false alarm rate was similar to that with real word stimuli, even with nonwords that did not resemble real words (see Parkin, Bindschaedler, & Squires, submitted, for a fuller account of these studies).

The last finding is hard to account for in terms of familiarity, as one would expect nonwords, which have never been encountered before, to have little in the way of familiarity. Recently Schacter, Curran, and Galluccio (1996) have reported similar findings in a frontal lobe patient BG. This patient, who suffered right frontal lobe damage, also produced high levels of false alarms, was insensitive to the associative overlap of distractors, and made high levels of false alarms to nonwords. To account for BG's impairment they suggested that he had a *focused retrieval deficit* in that when attempting to identify targets his criterion amounts to little more than "I saw a bunch of words". As a result of this criterion a large number of distractors along with targets are accepted. In support of this idea Schacter et al. show that BG's disastrously high false alarm rate can be removed if the targets and distractors come from different categories—thus, even though his retrieval criterion is poor it is sufficient to allow correct rejection of distractors (e.g. "everything I saw was from categories A,B,C not D,E,F").

Schacter et al.'s theory provides a good account of BG's recognition performance but does it account for, in the first instance, data from case JB? From the foregoing it is clear that many of the findings from BG are replicated in case JB and, indeed, a second case (MR; Parkin & Squires, in prep.) provides a further example. However, there are some difficulties in particular in explaining JB's performance on the abstract designs test. One could, as Schacter et al. have done, suggest that the ND/D manipulation is analogous to the studied/non-studied category manipulation, but there is a problem with this. In the category manipulation the distinction between studied and non-studied categories is transparent, easily verbalised, and not difficult to remember. In our ND/D manipulation there is no transparency concerning the features comprising the two stimulus sets; they are not easily verbalised, and extremely hard to remember. Thus it is difficult to see how they could coalesce into a retrieval criterion. Instead one must argue that it is the basic familiarity/unfamiliarity of the elements that allows recognition to occur. Thus, for JB at least, perceptual familiarity does affect his recognition memory, under certain conditions.

A second problem relates to patient ROB (Hanley, Davies, Downes, & Mayes, 1994; Hanley & Davies, this volume). As we saw, these authors argue that ROB's poor recall but good recognition should be interpreted within Shallice's (1988) framework, which proposes dissociable description and verification aspects of executive memory function. Thus ROB performs poorly on recall because she cannot provide effective descriptions, but has unimpaired recognition because verification processes are intact. Norman and Schacter (1996) have argued that the distinction made between description and verification cannot be sustained because the information providing the description cannot be operationally distinguished from that underlying verification, i.e. in verifying a target as correct, one must have retrieved information about the learning episode in order to know that the generated response is correct. Norman and Schacter go on to suggest that focused retrieval can undergo either partial breakdown—resulting in the patterns shown by BG and JB, or a complete breakdown in which familiarity alone serves to facilitate recognition. As Hanley and Davies point out, this leads to the rather implausible suggestion that ROB's excellent recognition memory, including that involving contextually demanding situations, is based solely on familiarity.

An important issue is whether the deficits observed in these patients are occurring at encoding or retrieval. As we have seen, Hanley and Davies have provided evidence that ROB's deficit is at retrieval on the grounds that she shows no improvement when encoding manipulations are used. Schacter et al.'s account is framed in terms of a retrieval deficit, but they do not offer any direct evidence to support this claim. However, their view gains support from recent PET studies, which have consistently associated right frontal function with episodic retrieval processes (e.g. Fletcher et al., 1995; Tulving et al., 1994).

We have recently examined the locus of JB's deficit by examining how factors affecting retrieval and encoding affect his recognition memory (Parkin et al., submitted). In studies employing a financial incentive to respond more accurately, we have found that this either increases false alarms or has no effect. Instructions to respond accurately by allowing JB to make only the same number of yes responses as there are targets also failed to reduce the proportion of false alarms. In contrast to this, manipulations of encoding do have a marked effect on JB. Figure 7.5 shows the results of a study in which JB either studied targets under free learning conditions or made a semantic orienting decision about each item. Although JB's false alarm rate remains elevated it is markedly reduced when encoding instructions are given.

We have argued that JB's memory impairment stems essentially from poor encoding. This results in a poor event description which, in turn, serves as an impoverished basis for constructing an effective retrieval context. As a result he is reliant on only a superficial representation of target information, which is sufficient to allow accurate target identification but at the cost of allowing

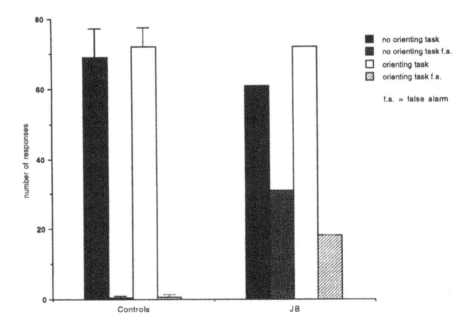

FIG. 7.5. Performance of JB and controls following semantic orienting task instructions or free learning.

many distractor items to be identified as well—thus, only when total dissimilarity between targets and distractors is achieved will JB's recognition memory be normal. Locating JB's deficit at the encoding stage also accounts for JB's highly defective recall (Parkin et al., 1996) and is consistent with PET studies showing left frontal activation during episodic learning (Fletcher et al., 1995; Tulving et al., 1994). Interestingly case MR (Parkin & Squires, in prep.) also responds markedly to the encoding manipulation and he also has a left-sided lesion.

Finally, why should JB be so poor at encoding? At present we do not know, but one possibility is that he attends rather broadly but at a very shallow level thus making him as likely to encode irrelevant detail as the main theme of an episode. An anecdote about JB does, however, suggest that there may be some truth in this idea. I recently accompanied JB to a "Holiday on Ice" show. This was an extravagant event centred on magic and was full of events such as levitation, vanishing women, and motorbike stunts. Throughout the performance he persistently nudged me and whispered a number such as "35". I thought nothing of this until next day when I asked him what the show had been about. "Well," he reflected, "I can tell you that there was one spotlight that didn't work and that the maximum number of dancers on the stage was 35".

"But what was the show about?"

He looked blank.

REFERENCES

Benton, A.L., & Hamsher, K.D. (1976). *Multilingual aphasia examination.* Iowa City: University of Iowa.

Eslinger, P.J., & Grattan, L.M. (1993). Frontal lobe and frontal-striatal substrates for different forms of human cognitive flexibility. *Neuropsychologia, 31*(1), 17–28.

Fletcher, P.C., Frith, C.D., Grasby, P.M., Shallice, T., Frackowiak, R.S.J., & Dolan, R.S.J. (1995). Brain systems for encoding and retrieval of auditory verbal memory. *Brain, 118,* 401–416.

Gardiner, J.M. & Java, R.I. (1992). Recognizing and remembering. In A. Collins, M.A. Conway, S.E. Gathercole, & P.E. Morris (Eds.), *Theories of Memory.* Hove, UK: Lawrence Erlbaum Associates Ltd.

Guildford, J.P., Christensen, P.R., Merrifield, P.R., & Wilson, R. (1978). *Alternate uses: Manual of instructions and interpretation.* Orange, CA: Sheridan Psychological Services.

Hanley, J.R., Davies, A.D.M., Downes, J.J., & Mayes, A.R. (1994). Impaired recall of verbal material following rupture and repair of an anterior communicating artery aneurysm. *Cognitive Neuropsychology, 11,* 543–578.

Harlow, J.M. (1993). Recovery from the passage of an iron bar through the head. *History of Psychiatry, 4,* 271–281. (Originally published 1868).

Nelson, H.E. (1976). A modified card sorting test sensitive to frontal lobe deficits. *Cortex, 12,* 313–324.

Nelson, H.E. (1985). *National Adult Reading Test.* London: NFER-Nelson.

Norman, K.A. & Schacter, D.L. (1996). Implicit memory, explicit memory and false recollection: A cognitive neuroscience perspective. To appear in L.M. Reder (Ed), *Implicit Memory and metacognition.* Hillsdale, NJ: Lawrence Erlbaum Associates Inc.

Parkin, A.J., Bindschaedler, C., Harsent, L., & Metzler, C. (1996). Pathological false alarm rates following damage to the left frontal cortex. *Brain and Cognition, 31*, 14–27.

Parkin, A.J., Bindschaedler, C., & Squires, E. (submitted). High false alarm rates following left frontal lesions: Further investigation and an explanation.

Parkin, A.J., & Leng, N.R.C. (1993). *Neuropsychology of the amnesic syndrome*. Hove, UK: Lawrence Erlbaum Associates Ltd.

Parkin, A.J., Leng, N.R.C., Stanhope, N., & Smith, A.L. (1988). Memory impairment following ruptured aneurysm of the anterior communicating artery. *Brain and Cognition, 7*, 231–243.

Parkin, A.J., & Squires, E.J. (in prep). Phenomenal misidentification due to left frontal lobe disease.

Raven, J.C. (1960). *Guide to the Standard Progressive Matrices*. London: H.K. Lewis.

Rey, A. (1964). *L'examen clinique en psychologie*. Paris: Presse Universitaires de France.

Ruff, M., Light, R.H., & Evans, R.W. (1987). The Ruff figural fluency test: A normative study with adults. *Developmental Neuropsychology, 3*, 37–51.

Schacter, D.L., Curran, T., & Galluccio, L. (1996). False recognition and the right frontal lobe. *Neurospychologia*, 793–808.

Shallice, T. (1988). *From neuropsychology to mental structure*. New York: Cambridge University Press.

Shallice, T., & Evans, M.E. (1978). The involvement of the frontal lobes in cognitive estimation, *Cortex, 14*, 294–303.

Trenerry, M.R., Crosson, B., DeBoe, J., & Leber, W.R. (1989). *Stroop Neuropsychological Screening Test*. Odessa, Fl: Psychological Assessment Resources.

Tulving, E. (1985). Memory and consciousness. *Canadian Psychologist, 26*, 1–12.

Tulving, E., Kapur, S., Craik, F.I.M., Moscovitch, M., & Houle, S. (1994). Hemispheric encoding/retrieval asymmetry in episodic memory: Positron emission tomography findings. *Proceedings of the National Academy of Sciences, USA, 91*, 2016–2020.

Warrington, E.K. (1984). *Recognition Memory Test*. London: NFER-Nelson.

Wechsler, D. (1981). *Wechsler Adult Intelligence Scale–Revised*. New York: Psychological Corporation.

Wechsler, D. (1984). *Wechsler Memory Scale–Revised*. New York: Psychological Corporation.

8 Schizophrenic Amnesia

Peter J. McKenna
Fulbourn Hospital, Cambridge and Department of Experimental Psychology, University of Cambridge, UK

Keith Laws
Psychology Department, University of Hertfordshire, Hatfield, UK

INTRODUCTION

When one thinks of amnesia, one usually thinks of disorders where there is focal neurological damage—to the hippocampus, mammillary bodies, thalamus or other structures—which cause memory impairment as their chief symptom. One might also think of general dementing disorders like Alzheimer's disease and Huntington's disease, as well as states of static diffuse brain damage, in which memory is affected as part of a wider pattern of poor cognitive performance. One does not, however, immediately make a connection with psychiatric illness, although, after some thought, it might be recalled that there are states of psychogenic amnesia, that patients with depression often complain of poor memory, and that, to a much lesser extent, memory has also been studied in other disorders such as anxiety.

Until recently, however, memory was not considered a serious topic of investigation in a further psychiatric disorder, schizophrenia. Such patients (unlike those with depression) rarely if ever complain of poor memory, and their relatives and carers do not as a rule comment on memory failures in everyday life. Nor do the symptoms of schizophrenia—delusions, hallucinations, incoherence of speech, emotional changes, social withdrawal, and occupational decline—seem to be even remotely related to memory or amnesia. Indeed, as a "functional" psychosis, schizophrenia should not be expected to be associated with any compromise of intellectual function whatsoever—this is the hallmark feature of "organic" psychoses like delirium and dementia.

To understand why memory is a legitimate topic of study in schizophrenia, one that has been neglected but is now a focus of considerable research interest, it is necessary to dip briefly into the history of thinking about the nature of the disorder. This has been characterised above all by a dispute that has been fought out over the century since schizophrenia was identified by Kraepelin in 1896, and which remains, to date, unresolved. One side in this dispute has been psychodynamic psychiatry—the followers of Freud who have always passionately believed that schizophrenia is psychologically determined; the result of unconscious conflicts or abnormal family dynamics. Any hint of organicity, of brain dysfunction in schizophrenia was—and is—anathema to this school of thought. The other side consists of those, beginning with Kraepelin, who called schizophrenia dementia praecox, who have always firmly believed that the disorder will ultimately be proved to be a biological brain disease, albeit one that is more subtle than the crude destructive processes seen in neurological disease.

For decades, particularly in America, the psychodynamic school of thought held sway. It began to falter when the first antipsychotic drug, chlorpromazine, was introduced in 1952 and quickly proved to be of substantial therapeutic benefit. Then, as evidence failed to materialise that schizophrenia can be precipitated by stressful life events (e.g. Day, 1981) or is related in any way to abnormal family interactions (see Hirsch & Leff, 1975), and in the face of accumulating evidence for a genetic factor (see Gottesman, 1991), the biological school of thought began to gain ground and is now the dominant force motivating research.

Completely incompatible with psychodynamic approaches (and more than a little unpalatable for psychiatry in general) is the idea that schizophrenia might be accompanied by the development of intellectual impairment. Yet, from the earliest psychological studies, it was invariably found that schizophrenic patients as a group showed a tendency to perform poorly on any cognitive task given to them (see Chapman & Chapman, 1973). Somewhat later, as intelligence testing became popular, schizophrenic patients were found to have lower IQs than the rest of the population—markedly so in the most severe cases—with at least some of the impairment being due to decline after the onset of illness (Payne, 1973). Next, three reviews examining the ability of neuro-psychological tests to distinguish schizophrenic patients from those with organic brain disease (Goldstein, 1978; Heaton, Baade, & Johnson, 1978; Malec, 1978) all concluded that it was impossible to do so for chronic schizophrenic patients. Ultimately, Crow and co-workers (Liddle & Crow, 1984; Owens & Johnstone, 1980; Stevens, Crow, Bowman, & Coles, 1978) demonstrated beyond reasonable doubt that among the most severely ill, chronically hospitalised schizophrenic patients something essentially indistinguishable from dementia supervenes in a minority of cases.

In the last 10 years there has been an explosion of interest in the neuropsychology of schizophrenia. As part of this, memory has been found to be an important area of deficit, which seems to stand out from the general tendency to poor performance. Furthermore, the pattern of impairment across the various domains of memory is emerging as being quite heterogeneous, and so is of considerable interest to neuropsychologists with their traditional emphasis on dissociations. Finally, there are strong suggestions that schizophrenic memory impairment extends into the domain of semantic memory, which marks it out from most other forms of memory disorder and which might conceivably be relevant to the understanding of some of the key symptoms of the disorder.

This chapter describes a patient who deviates considerably from the standard accounts of schizophrenia as described in psychiatric textbooks. She is, however, typical of the clinical picture of chronic, severe schizophrenia and provides an unexceptional example of the large number of so-called institutionalised patients. She also shows, in particularly marked form, the range of cognitive deficits that have recently been documented in schizophrenia, and these include what is emerging as a typical pattern of memory deficits.

SR: A PATIENT WITH CHRONIC, SEVERE SCHIZOPHRENIA

SR is a 53-year-old woman. As a child, she was described as lonely, introverted, and prone to phobias. Otherwise her childhood was unremarkable. She attended grammar school, but left at the age of 16 after failing her exams. At the age of 14 she started to complain increasingly about fears of dogs and long corridors; this was attributed to "normal adolescent difficulties". Between the ages of 16 and 17, while she was at secretarial college, she became increasingly withdrawn and seemed unable to concentrate or do anything for herself. She was also noted to "walk around in a daze". During this period she expressed the belief that her food was being poisoned.

She was first admitted to hospital in 1960 at the age of 18. Over the next two years she had a succession of admissions lasting a few days or a few weeks—typically she would insist on being discharged or would abscond home and refuse to return—until, by the age of 20, she was spending most of her time as an in-patient or attending as a day patient. The case notes at this time record her complaints of anxiety and depression, note her various phobias, and occasionally refer in passing to the fact that her manner was agitated and odd. Mainly, however, they are replete with references to what was considered to be SR's "highly pathogenic family situation". It was observed that "her main complaints concerned her ambivalent feelings towards her mother", who was seen as "a powerful destroying figure". She was considered to be "locked in bitter conflict with her parents as a duo". It was felt that the only hope for her was "to try and have a number of family conferences"; but doubts were expressed about this course of action as "there is considerable resistance to this ... both sides being afraid that their manoeuvring will be uncovered". SR's frequent relapses and re-admissions were sometimes explicitly attributed to the behaviour and attitudes of her parents.

Although no schizophrenic symptoms were recorded in SR's case notes during this period, a diagnosis of schizophrenia was nevertheless made. For the next 10 years she and her parents received, in line with the fashion of the time, family therapy. At first, there were regular intensive sessions with her parents, but later these became merely what were described as monthly family meetings. In addition, with little comment, SR was treated with a variety of different antipsychotic drugs.

Family therapy and drug treatment continued, but ultimately SR's parents found it increasingly difficult to cope with her behaviour. This included staying up all night, taking long walks in the rain, becoming distressed for no apparent reason, burning paper and sanitary towels in the living room, and once, when her parents went away for the weekend, letting the house deteriorate into a terrible state. In 1975, at the age of 33 and after over 15 years of illness, SR became permanently hospitalised.

SR's condition has remained much the same over the last 20 years. She presents as unkempt and her appearance is neglected, with long bedraggled grey hair. She is often to be seen wandering around the grounds, sometimes barefoot and in nightclothes, oblivious to her state and the weather. Most of the time she is not behaviourally disturbed, but can be noticed performing occasional odd, ritualistic behaviour, such as bowing in front of the ward clock. Every so often, however, she has periods lasting days or weeks at a time during which she becomes quite agitated, paces, runs up and down corridors, and storms about, screaming and engaging in behaviours like throwing her clothes away.

Outside periods of agitation, during which she rambles incoherently, SR's speech is easy to follow, but is hesitant, mechanical, and repetitive. She also shows so-called stilted speech, being excessively polite and formal at all times; for example, when being interviewed she typically thanks all the people in the room after each question, and when referring to her parents, calls them "Mr. and Mrs. F.A.W. R—"; once during a testing session involving naming pictures of famous people she insisted on giving each member of the royal family their full title, e.g. "her Royal Highness, Madam Princess Diana, the Princess Royal, Princess Diana".

When questioned about her mood SR will invariably state that she is unhappy, and full of bitterness and regrets about the way her life has turned out. Objectively, though, she does not seem depressed, only placid and somewhat remote. She also shows many features of schizophrenic emotional disorder:

generally she shows little expression of emotion ("affective flattening"), but from time to time, often for no reason, will break into a caricature of a polite smile ("inappropriate affect"). During states of agitation, she weeps and wails and appears distraught, even tormented, but moves quickly to laughter and back again. Like many schizophrenic patients, even when at her most distressed, her unhappiness seems somehow to lack depth or conviction.

On questioning about abnormal beliefs, SR will usually state that her brother is torturing her in unspecified ways, and that the hospital is planning to burn her. She has also expressed the idea that she has the gift of second sight and that she has a photographic memory (which, as will be seen, is very far from the truth). She also repeatedly alludes to the royal family; this almost certainly reflects a system of delusions about them, the exact content of which, however, is obscure. She intermittently experiences auditory hallucinations, hearing the voices of members of her family talking about torture and death, and that of the Queen reprimanding her. The voices sometimes tell her to what to do and have instructed her not to take her medication.

On casual examination, SR's cognitive status is intact. Like the vast majority of schizophrenic patients, she is oriented in time, although she sometimes gets the date wrong, and she knows the details of her surroundings, the names of staff, the ward, the hospital, and so on. Beyond this, however, vagueness creeps into her answers to questions about how long she has been in hospital, how long on this particular ward, which ward she was on before, and the names of doctors and nurses who previously looked after her. She has no real idea about current events in the world, or what is happening on television programmes that she watches. On a commonly used screening test for cognitive impairment, the Mini-Mental State Examination (Folstein, Folstein, & McHugh, 1975), she scored 25 out of a maximum of 30, which is just above the cut-off of 23/24 established for mild dementia.

SR's current IQ, as measured using the WAIS, is 93. In illnesses that are associated with intellectual decline, an estimate of an individual's best level of IQ functioning can be made using the National Adult Reading Test (NART) of Nelson (1982). This examines the ability to pronounce words such as *depot*, *thyme*, and *prelate* which do not follow the rules of English pronunciation. Being able to pronounce a word is a good index that its meaning was once known and this tends to be preserved even after knowledge of the meaning is lost. SR's estimated pre-illness IQ is 105 on this test, 12 points higher than her current WAIS IQ, but within the normal range of variation between the two tests of −16 to +21 points. Her pattern of WAIS performance, however, reveals a verbal IQ of 106 and a performance IQ of 76; such a large discrepancy would normally be considered highly suggestive of intellectual impairment.

A more detailed picture of SR's neuropsychological functioning can be built up from a range of standard tests she has been administered as part of a number of studies in which she has taken part.

146 Mckenna AND LAWS

Visual Perception

SR's performance on a range of visual perceptual tests was examined using the Visual Object and Space Perception (VOSP) battery of Warrington and James (1991). It can be seen from Table 8.1 that she performed normally on some tests, in particular those requiring basic figure–ground identification—for example detecting shapes against a degraded background and identifying letters with incomplete outlines. She also did well on tasks tapping simple visuospatial skills—for example determining whether a dot is in the centre of a square or not. On tasks involving higher levels of perceptual processing, in particular form perception, however, SR showed poor performance: on the Object Decision Test, which requires the subject to decide which of four silhouette shapes is a real object rather than an imaginary one, she scored just below a 5th percentile cut- off for impairment. On the Silhouettes Test, which in addition to recognising objects presented in silhouette requires their identification, she scored well in the impaired range.

SR's performance on other visual perceptual tasks followed a similar patchy pattern. Her attempt to copy the Rey–Osterrieth figure (Osterrieth, 1944) is shown in Fig. 8.1. It is clear that she made a creditable attempt at a quite arduous and time-consuming task, although her score, at 27 out of a maximum of 36, fell just outside the normal range (using a cut-off of two standard deviations below

TABLE 8.1
SR' s Performance on Tests of Visual and Visuospatial Function

Test	SR's score	Normal Score Range	Comment
Visual Object and Space Perception Battery			
Shape detection	20/20	18–20	Normal
Incomplete letters	19/20	10–20 5% cut-off 16	Normal
Object decision	13/20	12–20 5% cut-off 14	Minimally impaired
Silhouettes	9/30	13–30 5% cut-off 15	Impaired
Dot counting	10/10	9–10 5% cut-off 8	Normal
Position discrimination	19/20	15–20 5% cut-off 18	Normal
Other tests			
Rey figure copy	27/36	32 ± 2	Mildly impaired
Unusual views test	16/20	18–20	Impaired
Benton face matching test	27/54	41–54	Severely impaired

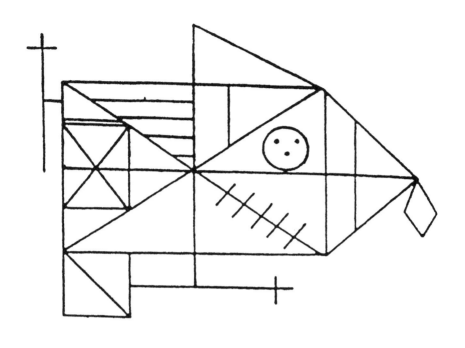

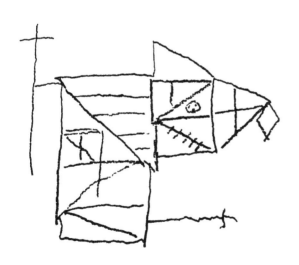

FIG. 8.1.   SR's copying of the Rey–Osterrieth figure.

the mean of 32 for normal adults). She was also mildly impaired on a task of form perception, the Unusual Views Test of Warrington and Taylor (1973), which requires photographs of objects taken from unconventional angles to be identified; she scored 16 out of 20 on this test, the cut-off for normals being 18. SR showed more evidence of impairment, however, on another task involving face processing: the Benton Face Matching test (Benton, Hamsher, Varney, & Spreen, 1978), which requires subjects to match the identity of faces photographed from different angles and under different lighting conditions. SR performed very poorly, scoring 27 out of a maximum of 54, when the cut-off for abnormality is 41.

Language

SR's performance on language tests is shown in Table 8.2. On a standard test of receptive syntactical competence, the Modified Token Test (De Renzi & Faglioni, 1978), she performed almost perfectly, being able to carry out increasingly grammatically complex instructions ranging from "Touch a circle" to "Instead of the white square, touch the yellow circle". Her performance on a variety of tests of expressive language competence, taken from two standard aphasia batteries (Kervetz, 1982; Schuell & Sefer, 1973), was also normal or only minimally impaired. Thus, she was able to repeat a series of 15 words and phrases ranging from *Sixty two and a half* to *Pack my box with five dozen jugs of*

TABLE 8.2
SR's Performance on Language Tests

Test	SR's score	Normal Score Range	Comment
Syntactic Modified Token Test	34/36	22–36 5% cut-off 28	Normal
Semantic Graded Naming Test	9/30	5–30 5% cut-off 13	Impaired for current verbal IQ level
Expressive Repetition of phrases*	99/100	–	Presumptively normal
Answering Simple Questions+	8/8	All normal controls scored 8	Normal
Producing Sentences+	6/6	All normal controls scored 6	Normal
Describing picture+	3 (1 = normal, 6= very impaired)	All normal controls scored 1	Impaired

*Western Aphasia Battery, +Minnesota Aphasia Battery

liquid veneer, making only one error. When given single words such as *coat* or *belongs*, she could produce correct and sensible sentences incorporating them.

On other language tests, however, she performed poorly. Her ability to describe a picture showing a house with people in the foreground carrying out activities like flying a kite and climbing a tree consisted only of a list of single words and brief phrases "Kite flying ... People pointing ... Smoke ... Chimney Man ... Tree ... Man searching ... House". This pattern of responding is very different from that of normal individuals, who invariably provide an integrated and well-formed narrative account. On a standard naming task, the Graded Naming Test (McKenna & Warrington, 1984), which requires the subject to name pictures of increasingly obscure animals and objects, SR scored 9 out of 30, lower than expected performance on the basis of both her estimated premorbid IQ and her current WAIS vocabulary score; in fact, her score is well below the 5th percentile cut-off for a population of 400 normal adults (P. McKenna, unpublished data). She named a kangaroo as a hare, handcuffs as cufflinks, a turtle as a water vole, and an anteater as a beaver.

To explore SR's naming difficulty further, she was asked to name the entire corpus of 260 line drawings of Snodgrass and Vanderwart (1980). She made 83 errors (see Table 8.3); the majority of these took the form of either semantic category errors (e.g. *accordion* for *trumpet*, *elephant* for *rhinoceros*) or giving the superordinate semantic category rather than the word itself (e.g. *musical instrument* for *trumpet*, *vegetable* for *asparagus*); however, she also produced some perseverative errors (many animals were named as *beaver*) and errors based on what seemed to be perceptual confusions (e.g. *anchor*→"Cross bones, like skull and cross bones"; *peanut*→"marrow"). Some of these errors are shown in Table 8.3. A multiple regression analysis showed that, although SR's naming was significantly influenced by item familiarity and name frequency, the visual complexity of items was unrelated to performance. This suggests that SR's naming deficit does not stem from a primary visual-perceptual problem. Intriguingly, a breakdown of SR's errors showed that she was worse at naming items from living (56% correct) than non-living (83% correct) categories.

Executive Function

Executive or frontal tests require one or more of the elements of decision making, selection of strategies, and ongoing checking and evaluation of responding, abilities that are at least partly mediated by the frontal lobes. The prototypical executive test is the Wisconsin Card Sorting Test, which requires subjects to sort cards with various designs according to rules that have to be worked out by trial and error and which change from time to time. Even using a simplified version of the task, where the subject is told when rule changes occur (Nelson, 1976), SR performed extremely poorly: although she grasped the initial sorting principle immediately, when this was changed she had great difficulty

TABLE 8.3
Some Examples of SR's Naming Errors

Cap–Shoe	Celery–Marrow	Chisel–Hammer	Duck–Pigeon	Guitar–Violin
Kangeroo–Camel	Nut–Screw	Rhino–Pig	Seal–Beaver	Squirrel–Fox
Tomato–Orange	Flute–Bagpipes	Lettuce–Cabbage	Lobster–Wasp	Nail File–Fountain Pen
Sheep–Beaver	Sledge–Stretcher	Alligator–Redcow	Bee–Locust	Fox–Dog
Orange–Peach	Peach–Plum	Screw–Nail	Anchor–Sleigh	Bat–Nail
Beetle–Fly	Cherry–Apple	French Horn–Accordion	Grapes–Leaf	Hammer–Chopper
Mitten–Funnel	Ostrich–Peacock	Penguin–Pelican	Roller Skate–Tricycle	Screwdriver–Matelot
Stove–Fridge	Ant–Blow fly	Donkey–Monkey	Monkey–Beaver	Peanut–Marrow
Pepper–Pumpkin	Sandwich–Double Bass	Sea-Horse–Water Nymph	Toe–Finger	Whistle–Calendar

adjusting her responding and made many perseverative errors. Ultimately she managed to achieve a score of two out of six categories; this contrasts with a 5th percentile cut-off of five categories for a group of 84 normal adults (McKenna et al., unpublished data).

Another widely used test that is sensitive to frontal function requires the subject to generate as many items in a category as possible in a specified time. SR did better on this task, naming 13 animals in one minute, a score that is just below the 5th percentile cut-off for the same group of 84 normal individuals. Another, quite different, executive task is the Cognitive Estimates Test of Shallice and Evans (1978). In this test, subjects have to make educated guesses about questions to which they would not normally know the exact answer; responses are scored from 0–3 according to their extremeness. SR scored 17 on this, estimating the speed at which racehorses gallop as 12mph and the length of an average man's spine as 40 feet. This score is well outside the fifth percentile cut-off of 13 for the above 84 normal individuals.

Memory

SR's memory was first tested using a relatively undemanding screening test, the Rivermead Behavioural Memory Test (RBMT) (Wilson, Cockburn, & Baddeley, 1985). This consists of 12 subtests, covering memory functions such as orientation, recall and recognition, remembering a route, plus tests of prospective memory (i.e. remembering to do things). Passing each of the subtests gives a score of 1, and most normal individuals score 10 or more. SR scored only 2 out of 12 on this test—this is in the "severely impaired" range, typically seen in patients with amnesia, dementia, or severe head injury.

The RBMT is a clinical test, which yields little information about the integrity of various different components of memory (although its subtests tap largely long-term memory). Further testing was therefore directed specifically to SR's performance on tests of short-term memory and different aspects of long-term memory.

Short-term memory holds around seven items of information for up to 30 seconds, and is typically tested by span tasks. The concept of short-term memory has been elaborated by Baddeley (1986) into that of working memory, a multi-component system that allows the performance of complex tasks like reading, comprehension, and mental arithmetic. SR's performance on standard span tests is shown in Table 8.4. Her digit span was 7 forwards and her performance on a non-verbal equivalent, the Corsi block tapping test, was 5; both scores are well within the normal range. One task that is believed to place demands on working memory is reverse digit span. However, at 6, SR's performance on this was at the 95th percentile for normal individuals. Another working memory task involves so-called dual task performance. In one example of such a test (Baddeley et al., 1997) subjects have to repeat series of digits at the upper limit of their span while simultaneously carrying out a second task of putting crosses in boxes. SR filled in 97 boxes in 2 minutes under single task conditions, and this dropped to 79 while simultaneously carrying out the digit span task. There was no change in her digit span performance under single and dual task conditions: she completed 14 spans of 5 digits under the single task condition, making 6 errors; under the dual task condition she completed 14 spans, making 5 errors. SR's dual task decrement (*mu*) score, which takes into account changes in performance on both components of the task, was 94%, once again well within the normal range.

SR's long-term memory was examined using the Doors and People Test, (Baddeley, Emslie, & Nimmo-Smith, 1994), which contains tests of verbal recall and recognition (recalling a series of four names of individuals and recognising 24 surnames out of sets of four), and visual recall and recognition (recalling four shapes and recognising 24 pictures of doors from sets of four), all

TABLE 8.4
SR's Short-term and Working Memory Performance

Test	SR's Score	Normal Score Range	Comment
Forward digit span	7	5 or more	Normal
Reverse digit span	6	3 or more	Superior
Corsi blocks	5	1 or 2 less than digit span	Normal
Dual task decrement (*mu*)	94%	54–120% (Median 91.4%)	Normal

of which are matched for difficulty. As can be seen from Table 8.5, in contrast to her short-term memory performance, SR was moderately or severely impaired on all four components of this test.

Semantic memory refers to our long-term store of knowledge: this ranges from knowledge about words (e.g. knowing the meaning of the word *generous*) and general knowledge (e.g. knowing the capital of France), to highly abstract concepts (e.g. what justice is) and the rules governing social behaviour (e.g. knowing not to order dessert along with the starter and main course in a restaurant). As there are strong suggestions from the testing of SR's visual perceptual and language function that she has particular difficulty with tasks requiring naming and identification of objects, her semantic memory was examined in more depth.

The most well-known semantic memory test is the Semantic Processing or "Silly Sentences" Test (Collins & Quillian, 1969; Baddeley et al., 1992), in which subjects have to verify 50 sentences like *Rats have teeth* and *Tractors grow in gardens*. The time taken is the usual measure of the integrity of semantic memory; errors are rarely made by normal subjects. SR was somewhat slow on an orally presented version of this task, taking an average of 4.2 seconds/sentence compared with a mean of 3.3±0.5 seconds/sentence for 44 normal subjects. She also made two errors, the maximum made by normal subjects. SR was then presented with an untimed version of a similar, but somewhat harder test (Laws, Humber, Ramsey, & McCarthy, 1995a), in which subjects have to verify statements expressing subject–attribute relationships; half of the statements are true and half are false, but none of the false statements are as absurd as those in the "Silly Sentences" test. SR made 11/56 errors, rejecting 2/28 true statements (e.g. *Snails have shells*) and accepting 9/28 false statements (e.g. *Hairbrushes have roofs*). This error frequency is well above the maximum for 45 normal control subjects (mean total error rate = 4.06±1.98).

Two more tests underline the difficulties that SR has with tasks that require elementary semantic knowledge. In the first, she was presented with a lexical-decision task comprising 10 real and 10 non-real words in random order on a sheet of paper. All of the real words were high frequency and the non-words were matched to the real words for length. She was unable to discriminate between real

TABLE 8.5
SR's Long-term Memory Performance (Doors and People Test)

Test	SR's Score	Normal Score Range	Comment
Verbal recall	2/36	7–36 (5% cut-off 16)	Severely impaired
Verbal recognition	11/24	9–23 (5% cut-off 13)	Impaired
Visual recall	7/36	5–36 (5% cut-off 23)	Impaired
Visual recognition	9/24	8–24 (5% cut-off 13)	Impaired

and non-real words and identified all 20 words as real. In the second test, she was read aloud pairs of words, some of which were synonyms while other were unrelated. She was unable to judge synonyms above the level expected by chance.

Non-verbal semantic memory was also examined. The Object Decision Test (Humphreys & Riddoch 1987) requires subjects to classify drawings of real objects and "chimeras" (for example, made up by combining the head of one animal with the body of another) as real or imaginary. SR scored 36/64 on this test, which is barely above the chance level of 32. On the Pyramids and Palm Trees test (Howard & Patterson 1992), subjects are required to decide which of two alternative pictures (e.g. *palm tree* or *fir tree*) is related to a target object (e.g. *Egyptian pyramid*). SR scored 37/52, again not greatly above the chance level of 27, and well below the lower limit of performance by normal individuals of 49. SR's performance on these tasks shows that even when explicit verbal responses are not required, she has difficulty performing the kinds of semantic tasks that normals perform with ease.

A final area where semantic memory is important is in recognition of people. To examine this, SR was presented with 53 photographs of famous people from various eras and walks of life (e.g. *Marilyn Monroe, Nelson Mandela, Luciano Pavarotti*). She was encouraged to give their names and produce as much other identifying information as she could about each person, such as their occupations and why they were famous. Her scores are shown in Table 8.6. She managed to name only 9/53 faces and could provide the occupations for another six—this performance was severely impaired in comparison to 20 age- and IQ-matched normal controls. She was restricted to naming members of the royal family, Margaret Thatcher, and Adolf Hitler. Most of her other replies consisted of "don't know" responses, but she also made several stereotyped forename responses (e.g. *Saddam Hussein*→"At a guess, he could be called Lewis"; *Clint Eastwood*→"At a guess, he could be called Rupert").

TABLE 8.6
SR's Naming and Identification of Famous Faces

	SR	Normal controls (n=20)
Age	48	40±16.62
NART IQ	105	107.95± 8.86
Named	9*	39.6± 8.75
Specific Identification	10**	42.5± 8.51
General Identification	15***	44.8± 6.94

*z=<.001
**z=<.0004
***z=.0001

It could be argued that some or all of SR's face identification impairment may have been due to high-level perceptual difficulties, as she performed poorly on the Benton Face Matching test, as noted earlier. However, SR also performed poorly on tests requiring her to produce semantic information about famous people when given their names. She managed to identify (i.e. give occupations and other information about) only 6/10 very famous names, including *Charlie Chaplin, Bill Clinton, Saddam Hussein, John Major, Adolf Hitler, Elvis Presley,* and *Marilyn Monroe.* Given the "ceiling" performance of normal controls at identifying these 10 names, any failures at all are very notable.

DISCUSSION

Schizophrenia: Psychological Disturbance or Brain Disease?

SR's case illustrates the deep divisions that have run through psychiatric thinking about the nature of schizophrenia. She became ill when psychodynamic theories of schizophrenia were in their heyday and at that time she seemed to provide ample support for the view that pathological family relationships were the root cause of the disorder. Thirty years on, many would regard the profound destructive effects her illness has had on her personality and mental life, not to mention her cognitive function, as typifying why schizophrenia is currently considered to be a biological brain disease. The prolonged battle between biological and psychodynamic psychiatry over schizophenia has certainly left a legacy of ambivalence about its nature in the minds of many. So, for example, while Ron and Harvey (1990, p.725) stated confidently that "to have forgotten that schizophrenia is a brain disease will go down as one of the great medical aberrations of the twentieth century", one of the major figures in social psychiatric research, Brown (1985, p.8), recalled his early "revulsion at reading some of the standard psychiatric accounts of the condition" and just as confidently re-affirmed his belief that emotional factors were of major importance.

Ignoring both sides' propaganda, what is known with certainty about the cause of schizophrenia? There are only two findings that can be regarded as established beyond reasonable doubt. One is that the disorder shows a familial tendency, which a series of twin and adoption studies has shown to reflect the operation of a genetic factor rather than some pathological feature of the family environment of individuals who become schizophrenic (e.g. see Gottesman, 1991). Nevertheless, it is evident that the hereditary contribution to schizophrenia is not great: the concordance rate for monozygotic twins is only 50%, and around two-thirds of patients who become schizophrenic will have no affected relatives in their extended families. The other finding is that, as a group, schizophrenic patients have larger lateral ventricles than normal subjects.

Initially exaggerated and subsequently the subject of some negative findings (see Lewis, 1990; Van Horn & McManus, 1992), the reality of lateral ventricular enlargement in schizophrenia has been placed beyond reasonable doubt by two large and well-controlled studies (Andreasen et al., 1990; Jones, Harvey, Lewis, & Murray, 1994). The magnitude of the enlargement, however, is small and the overlap with the normal population is great; it may not be present in female schizophrenic patients; it is not clearly related to any clinical variable; and it is probably already present at the earliest stages of illness. Lateral ventricular enlargement may therefore best be regarded as a trait-marker or risk-factor for schizophrenia rather than some direct index of brain disease.

The role of non-biological factors in causing schizophrenia is, at best, minor. The evidence in favour of family theories, as reviewed by Hirsch and Leff (1975), has always been weak. After these authors themselves (Hirsch & Leff, 1971) failed to replicate the strongest finding in this area, of a deviant style of communication in the parents of schizophrenic patients, this line of investigation effectively came to a halt. As regards the role of stress, the majority of nine studies of life events preceding the onset of schizophrenia (see Bebbington & Kuipers, 1988; Bebbington, Bowen, Hirsch, & Kuipers, 1995), have failed to find any evidence for an excess of these. In particular, there is very little evidence from these studies to suggest that life events are a significant factor in precipitating a first episode of schizophrenia.

All other claims for abnormality in schizophrenia are uncertain. On the biological side, the fact that antipsychotic "neuroleptic" drugs are therapeutically effective (indeed, are the only treatment of proven effectiveness) provides strong circumstantial evidence for an underlying neurochemical abnormality. These drugs are known to exert their effect by blocking dopamine receptors. However, despite many ingenious attempts, no decisive evidence of a functional dopamine excess in the brains of schizophrenic patients has been forthcoming (see McKenna, 1994, for a review), and no other neurochemical abnormality has as yet been convincingly demonstrated. Beyond lateral ventricular enlargement, no structural abnormality has been firmly established in schizophrenia, but there are strong indications that there are both macroscopic and microscopic changes in the temporal lobes and its constituent structures like the hippocampus (for a review see Chua & McKenna, 1995). The leading claim for functional brain abnormality in schizophrenia has been so-called hypofrontality, a lowering of neuronal activity in the prefrontal cortex. However, hypofrontality has been found in only about a third of around 30 studies examining the brain under resting conditions, and claims for "activation" hypofrontality—i.e. failure to increase prefrontal activity during performance of an executive task—have also not been consistently supported (see Chua & McKenna, 1995; Gur & Gur 1995). It may be that schizophrenia is characterised by more subtle and complicated patterns of functional imaging abnormality, both at rest (Liddle et al., 1992) and with neuropsychological task activation (Frith et al., 1995), but these claims have not so far survived the test of replication.

On the psychological side, while stress does not seem to play any great role in causing schizophrenia in the first place, it is probably unwise to ignore such factors altogether. A number of early studies by Brown and co-workers (see Brown, 1985) suggested that the stress associated with living with relatives increases the risk of relapse in established illness. The important factors seemed to be high levels of negative emotional responses like criticism, hostility, and over-involvement on the part of the patients' relatives. Expressed emotion has gone on to become a large and productive area of schizophrenia research; in a review of 26 studies, Kavanagh (1992) found a significant association between high levels of expressed emotion and relapse in 16 of them.

The Neuropsychology of Schizophrenia

One of the most robust findings in schizophrenia research is that of wide-ranging cognitive impairment in the disorder. In the psychodynamically dominated period that lasted most of this century, this finding was, for the most part, studiously ignored. Even when it was acknowledged, typically by psychologists rather than psychiatrists, it was attributed to poor motivation and lack of co-operation, or to the interfering effects of psychotic symptoms. Thus in a well-known account, Chapman and Chapman (1973, p.34) stated, "To a large extent, lowered IQ test performance by schizophrenics reflects severity of pathology ... schizophrenics earn low IQ scores because they are disturbed rather than because they are dull". Later, it became a widely accepted, if tacit, policy to attribute poor neuropsychological test performance to treatment with neuroleptic drugs. This was despite the unanimous conclusion of many studies that drug treatment had little or no effect on most or all aspects of cognitive function in normal individuals—and if anything, tended to improve this in schizophrenic patients (e.g. King, 1990).

That schizophrenia is associated with the development of overall intellectual impairment that is largely a function of severity and chronicity of illness is now widely accepted (e.g. Frith, 1992; Goldberg & Gold, 1995). SR provides a typical example of the degree of impairment that is routinely encountered in chronically hospitalised patients. She is not demented in the usual sense of the term, being oriented and scoring in the normal range on the MMSE, albeit at the lower end of this. IQ testing, however, with a verbal–performance IQ discrepancy of over 30 points, does suggest that some degree of intellectual decline has taken place. In addition, more detailed neuropsychological testing reveals that she fails some tests in all domains of function.

As well as being associated with general intellectual impairment, it has been suggested that there are specific neuropsychological deficits in schizophrenia. Such impairments have been claimed in visual perception, for example in higher-level form perception and facial emotion processing, and also in all aspects of attention, and many aspects of language (see Cutting, 1985, for a review). Unfortunately it is unclear whether any of these are genuinely specific, in the sense of being disproportionate to the overall level of intellectual function, and perhaps the simplest explanation of the impairments that have been found in these areas is that they are merely examples of the general poor cognitive performance that characterises schizophrenia.

There may, however, be an exception in executive function. Virtually all studies (e.g. Goldberg et al., 1987; Kolb & Whishaw, 1983; Liddle & Morris, 1991; Morice, 1990) have found poor performance on tests of "frontal" function in schizophrenia. This has been found to be disproportionate to general intellectual impairment in some group studies (Crawford, Obonswain, & Bremner, 1993; Elliott, McKenna, Robbins, & Sahakian, 1995) but not in others (Braff et al., 1991; Saykin et al., 1991, 1994). However, an influential single case study by Shallice, Burgess, and Frith (1991) has provided persuasive support for a specific executive deficit in schizophrenia. They found that all of five chronically hospitalised patients showed a high frequency of impairment on a battery of 10 tests sensitive to frontal lobe lesions; in two patients this was against a background of general intellectual impairment, but in a further two it was relatively isolated; the remaining patient showed an intermediate pattern of performance.

SR also shows clear evidence of executive impairment. Against a background of mild or at most moderate general intellectual impairment, her performance on a range of standard executive tests ranges from the minimally impaired to the disastrous. In fact, her overall pattern of neuropsychological performance fits in well with that of Shallice et al.'s (1991) patients.

Another area of potential disproportionate deficit in schizophrenia is memory. Virtually all of around 30 studies reviewed by Cutting (1985) found some evidence of poor performance on memory tests in schizophrenia, and in chronic patients the impairment could be pronounced (Calev, 1984; Calev, Berlin, & Lerer, 1987). Subsequent studies have indicated that memory is commonly substantially impaired in schizophrenia. Thus McKenna et al. (1990) and Duffy and O'Carroll (1994) found that groups of schizophrenic patients designed to be representative of the disorder as a whole did not differ in their performance on the RBMT from a group of patients with head injury attending a rehabilitation centre. These and other studies have also suggested that memory impairment in schizophrenia is more marked than overall intellectual impairment (Gold, Randolph, & Carpenter, 1992; McKenna et al., 1990) and impairment in other domains of neuropsychological function (Saykin et al. 1991), although there have been a few conflicting findings (Blanchard & Neale, 1994; Saykin et al., 1994).

Whether or not it is specific in the sense of being disproportionate, memory impairment in schizophrenia certainly appears to be specific in another neuropsychological sense—that of showing a pattern of dissociations. The classical amnesic syndrome pattern of impaired long-term memory coupled with intact or relatively intact short-term memory has been highlighted in some recent studies (Duffy & O'Carroll, 1994; Tamlyn et al., 1992) and is also evident in others (e.g. Shallice et al., 1991; Goldberg et al., 1993). As with the classical amnesic syndrome, schizophrenic memory impairment has also been found to spare procedural and implicit memory (e.g. Clare, McKenna, Mortimer, & Baddeley, 1993; Goldberg et al., 1993), although the relevant studies are not unanimous on this point (see McKenna, Clare, & Baddeley, 1995 for a discussion).

SR conforms closely to this pattern: her short-term memory function appears to be well preserved in the face of long-term memory function that is at amnesic or demented levels. The sparing of short-term memory in her case also seems to encompass intact working memory, as probed by reverse digit span and dual task performance. This might be considered somewhat surprising in view of recent theoretical proposals that working memory, as an area of high-level integration of cognitive activity, is a good candidate for the locus of psychological abnormality in schizophrenia (Fleming, Goldberg, & Gold, 1994; Goldman-Rakic, 1991). Two studies (Fleming, Goldberg, Gold, & Weinberger, 1995; Park & Holzman, 1992) have in fact found indications of working memory impairment in schizophrenic patients. However, one further study comparing reverse digit span between schizophrenic patients and their non-schizophrenic monozygotic co-twins found only a trend to impairment (Goldberg et al., 1993).

Semantic Memory Impairment in Schizophrenia

Although memory impairment in schizophrenia seems to follow the pattern of the classical amnesic syndrome pattern quite closely, there appears to be one glaring difference. Semantic memory, memory for knowledge about the world, remains intact in the amnesic syndrome, at least for information acquired before the onset of amnesia (e.g. Squire, 1987), whereas in schizophrenia there is now a considerable body of evidence for widespread deficits that affect the most basic aspects of general knowledge. Perhaps the first suggestion of this was made by Cutting and Murphy (1988); they found that relatively young, acutely ill schizophrenic patients showed surprisingly poor performance on a test of knowledge about events and behaviour in the real world—this included questions about what to do with a large gambling win, and how to tell a friend they had overstayed their welcome. Subsequently, poor performance has been documented on the "Silly Sentences" test (Duffy & O'Carroll, 1994; Tamlyn et al., 1992) and other standard tasks (Clare et al., 1993; McKay et al., 1996). The last of these studies also provided preliminary evidence that the semantic memory deficit in schizophrenia is disproportionate to the overall level of intellectual impairment, and that it can sometimes be very pronounced—a group of elderly chronically hospitalised schizophrenic patients were found to perform no better than a group of patients with Alzheimer's disease on many of the subtests of a battery of semantic memory tests.

SR shows semantic memory deficits in marked, even spectacular form. This applies to both verbal and visual semantics and is present even on tasks that require no explicit retrieval of information. In some cases her knowledge about the world and people is virtually non-existent, in others it seems distorted. It cannot be stated that SR's semantic memory impairment is disproportionate to her overall level of intellectual impairment, and she shows quite marked deficits in areas, such as unfamiliar face matching, which require little if any semantic knowledge. Nevertheless, impairment on tests requiring access to semantic memory form a distinct, almost predictable theme running through her neuropsychological performance as a whole. Thus, in addition to poor performance on semantic memory tests *per se*, her language function shows a dissociation between impaired semantics and preserved syntax, and her visual perceptual performance shows that the most marked deficits are on tests such as naming silhouettes that require the accessing of semantic knowledge.

Similarities may be drawn between SR's pattern of naming performance and that in some neurological patients (often involving bilateral temporal lobe lesions) with category-specific semantic disorders (e.g. Gainotti, Silveri, Daniele, & Giustolisi, 1995), in that she shows a greater degree of impairment for naming living things as opposed to man-made objects. This differentially worse naming of animate items continued in sets matched for "nuisance" variables such as item familiarity and name frequency. Such findings in neurological patients have aroused considerable interest among neuropsychologists because they may provide information about the way semantic knowledge is organised (for example, by category or by attribute). Whether such a pattern does genuinely reflect the way in which the brain stores and organises knowledge remains to be fully established (Funnell & Sheridan, 1992; Stewart, Parkin, & Hunkin, 1992). Nevertheless, it is intriguing that schizophrenic patients may show a similar disorganisation or loss to their semantic knowledge base; in particular, the rarity and strangeness of such a disorder, if anything, only add to the psychological reality of this disorder in schizophrenic patients.

Another intriguing aspect of semantic memory impairment in schizophrenia is its potential relationship to symptoms. Although, as pointed out at the beginning of this chapter, poor memory performance in schizophrenia seems quite unconnected with the core features of the disorder, there might be more scope for accounting for schizophrenic symptoms like incoherence of speech, paranoia, and other delusions in terms of abnormal access to word meanings, disturbed knowledge about the world, breakdown and distortion of high-level concepts, and so on. Such an approach might seem speculative, but it is not, in fact, very dissimilar to that of a current leading theory of schizophrenic symptoms: Frith (1992) has argued that many schizophrenic symptoms can be understood in terms of a fundamental disorder of "second order" representations of knowledge about the world—knowledge which, like that held in semantic memory, is independent of personal experience.

Whatever the ultimate fate of theories of this type, it is evident that semantic memory is not related to schizophrenic symptoms in any simple way. Semantic memory impairment in schizophrenia has been found not to correlate with presence of delusions or hallucinations in schizophrenic patients (Tamlyn et al., 1992) or any other symptom for that matter (Chen, Wilkins, & McKenna, 1994; Duffy & O'Carroll, 1994). It is, however, possible that there may be more subtle relationships. For example, SR, whose delusions (and also her auditory hallucinations) involve royalty, named 7/7 (100%) of the members of the royal family but only 2/46 (4%) of the other faces (this differentially superior naming of royal family members is unlikely to reflect any greater familiarity of those faces, as the other faces also included many very famous people). This finding might be dismissed as a coincidence, except for the fact that a strikingly similar pattern has been documented in another patient, TG, by Laws, McKenna, and McCarthy (1995b). In the setting of severely impaired naming and identification of famous people, TG displayed a selective preservation of knowledge about political figures (particularly domestic politicians). His leading schizophrenic symptom consisted of grandiose delusions which were also mainly political—he believed that he was an MP and a friend of many prominent Conservatives.

In summary, SR and the many severe, chronic patients like her have been neglected in research, but they clearly have much to tell us about the nature of schizophrenia. At a clinical level, she shows the disorder in its true colours, not as a state characterised by the development of fascinating symptoms like delusions and hallucinations, but as a lifelong, crippling affliction, in which, in the words of Kraepelin (1913, p.74), "the essence of the personality is destroyed, the best and most precious part of its being torn from her". At a psychological level, cases like hers have established what is now widely accepted as the neuropsychological profile of schizophrenia: a disorder associated with a variable tendency to develop overall intellectual decline, superimposed on which are (probably) disproportionate deficits in memory and executive function. Although it is perhaps not seen in very sharp focus, SR's case in particular hints at the existence of a further specific deficit in schizophrenia—semantic memory impairment—which may ultimately turn out to have the theoretical power to begin to bridge the gulf between the neuropsychology and the extraordinary clinical phenomena of schizophrenia.

REFERENCES

Baddeley, A.D. (1986). *Working memory*. Oxford: Clarendon.
Baddeley, A.D., Della Sala, S., Gray, C., Papagno, C., & Spinnler, H. (1997). Testing central executive functioning with a pencil-and-paper test. In P. Rabbitt (Ed.), *Methodology of frontal and executive functions*. Hove, UK: Psychology Press.

Baddeley, A.D., Emslie, H., & Nimmo-Smith, I. (1992). *The Speed and Capacity of Language Processing (SCOLP) Test*. Bury St Edmunds, UK: Thames Valley Test Co.

Baddeley, A.D., Emslie, H., & Nimmo-Smith. I. (1994). *Doors and People: A test of visual and verbal recall and recognition*. Bury St Edmunds, UK: Thames Valley Test Co.

Bebbington, P.E., Bowen, J., Hirsch, S.R., & Kuipers, E.A. (1995). Schizophrenia and psychosocial stressors. In S.R. Hirsch & D.R. Weinberger (Eds.), *Schizophrenia*. Oxford: Blackwell.

Bebbington, P., & Kuipers, L. (1988). Social influences on schizophrenia. In P. Bebbington & P. McGuffin (Eds.), *Schizophrenia: The major issues*. Oxford: Heinemann/Mental Health Foundation.

Benton, A.L., Hamsher, K. de S., Varney, N.R., & Spreen, O. (1978). *Facial recognition*. New York: Oxford University Press.

Blanchard, J.J., & Neale, J.M. (1994). The neuropsychological signature of schizophrenia—generalized or differential deficit. *American Journal of Psychiatry, 151*, 40–48.

Braff, D.L., Heaton, R., Kuck, J., Cullum, M., Moranville, J., Grant, I., & Zisook, S. (1991). The generalised pattern of neuropsychological deficits in outpatients with chronic schizophrenia with heterogeneous Wisconsin Card Sorting Test results. *Archives of General Psychiatry, 48*, 891–898.

Brown, G.W. (1985). The discovery of expressed emotion: Induction or deduction? In J. Leff & C. Vaughn (Eds.), *Expressed emotion in families: Its significance for mental illness*. London: Guilford Press.

Calev, A. (1984). Recall and recognition in chronic nondemented schizophrenics: The use of matched tasks. *Journal of Abnormal Psychology, 93*, 172–177.

Calev, A., Berlin, H., & Lerer, B. (1987). Remote and recent memory in long-hospitalised chronic schizophrenics. *Biological Psychiatry, 22*, 79–85.

Chapman, L.J., & Chapman, J.P. (1973). *Disordered thought in schizophrenia*. New York: Appleton-Century-Crofts.

Chen, E.Y.H., Wilkins, A.J., & McKenna, P.J. (1994). Semantic memory is both impaired and anomalous in schizophrenia. *Psychological Medicine, 24*, 193–202.

Chua, S.E., & McKenna, P.J. (1995). Schizophrenia—A brain disease? A critical review of structural and functional cerebral abnormality in the disorder. *British Journal of Psychiatry, 166*, 563–582.

Clare, L., McKenna, P.J., Mortimer, A.M., & Baddeley, A.D. (1993). Memory in schizophrenia: What is impaired and what is preserved? *Neuropsychologia, 31*, 1225–1241.

Collins, A.M., & Quillian, M.R. (1969). Retrieval time from semantic memory. *Journal of Verbal Learning and Verbal Behavior, 8*, 240–247.

Crawford, J.R., Obonswain, M.C., & Bremner, M. (1993). Frontal lobe impairment in schizophrenia: Relationship to intellectual functioning. *Psychological Medicine, 23*, 787–790.

Cutting, J. (1985). *The psychology of schizophrenia*. Edinburgh: Churchill Livingstone.

Cutting, J., & Murphy, D. (1988). Schizophrenic thought disorder: A psychological and organic interpretation. *British Journal of Psychiatry, 152*, 310–319.

Day, R. (1981). Life events and schizophrenia: The "triggering" hypothesis. *Acta Psychiatrica Scandinavica, 64*, 97–122.

De Renzi, E., & Faglioni, P. (1978). Normative data and screening power of a shortened version of the Token Text. *Cortex, 14*, 41–49.

Duffy, L., & O'Carroll, R. (1994). Memory impairment in schizophrenia—A comparison with that observed in the alcoholic Korsakoff syndrome. *Psychological Medicine, 24*, 155–166.

Elliott, R., McKenna, P.J., Robbins, T.W., & Sahakian, B.J. (1995). Neuropsychological evidence for fronto-striatal dysfunction in schizophrenia. *Psychological Medicine, 25*, 619–630.

Fleming, K., Goldberg, T.E., & Gold, J.M. (1994). Applying working memory constructs to schizophrenic cognitive impairment. In A.S. David & J.C. Cutting (Eds.), *The neuropsychology of schizophrenia.* Hove, UK: Lawrence Erlbaum Associates Ltd.

Fleming, K., Goldberg, T.E., Gold, J.M., & Weinberger, D.R. (1995). Verbal working memory dysfunction in schizophrenia: Use of a Brown-Peterson paradigm. *Psychiatry Research, 56,* 155–161.

Folstein, M.F., Folstein, S.E., & McHugh, P.R. (1975). 'Mini-Mental State': A practical method for grading the cognitive state of patients for the clinician. *Journal of Psychiatric Research, 12,* 189–198.

Frith, C.D. (1992). *The cognitive neuropsychology of schizophrenia.* Hove, UK: Lawrence Erlbaum Associates Ltd.

Frith, C.D., Friston, K.J., Herold, S., Silbersweig, D., Fletcher, P., Cahill, C., Dolan, R.J., Frackowiak, R.S.J., & Liddle, P.F. (1995). Regional brain activity in chronic schizophrenic patients during the performance of a verbal fluency task. *British Journal of Psychiatry, 167,* 343–349.

Frith, C.D., Leary, J., Cahill, C., & Johnstone, E.C. (1991). IV. Performance on psychological tests. Demographic and clinical correlates of the tests. *British Journal of Psychiatry, 159,* supplement 13, 26–29.

Funnell, E., & Sheridan, J. (1992). Categories of knowledge? Unfamiliar aspects of living and nonliving things. *Cognitive Neuropsychology, 9,* 135–153.

Gainotti, G., Silveri, M.C., Daniele, A., & Giustolisi, L. (1995). Neuroanatomical correlates of category-specific semantic disorders: A critical survey. *Memory, 3,* 247–264.

Gold, J.M., Randolph, C., & Carpenter, C.J. (1992). The performance of patients with schizophrenia on the Wechsler Memory Scale–Revised. *Clinical Neuropsychologist, 6,* 367–370.

Goldberg, T.E., & Gold, J.M. (1995). Neurocognitive deficits in schizophrenia. In S.R. Hirsch & D.F. Weinberger (Eds.), *Schizophrenia.* Oxford: Blackwell.

Goldberg, T.E., Torrey, E.F., Gold, J.M., Ragland, J.D., Bigelow, L.B., & Weinberger, D.R. (1993). Learning and memory in monozygotic twins discordant for schizophrenia. *Psychological Medicine, 23,* 71–85.

Goldberg, T.E., Weinberger, D.R., Berman, K.F., Pliskin, N.H., & Podd, M.H. (1987). Further evidence for dementia of prefrontal type in schizophrenia? A controlled study of teaching the Wisconsin Card Sorting Test. *Archives of General Psychiatry, 44,* 1008–1014.

Goldman-Rakic, P.S. (1991). Prefrontal cortical dysfunction in schizophrenia: the relevance of working memory. In B.J. Carroll & J.E. Barrett (Eds.), *Psychopathology and the brain,* New York: Raven Press.

Goldstein, G. (1978). Cognitive and perceptual differences between schizophrenics and organics. *Schizophrenia Bulletin, 4,* 160–185.

Gottesman, I.I. (1991). *Schizophrenia genesis: The origins of madness.* New York: Freeman.

Gur, R.C., & Gur, R.E. (1995). Hypofrontality in schizophrenia: RIP. *Lancet, i,* 1383–1384.

Heaton, R.K., Baade, L.E., & Johnson, K.L. (1978). Neuropsychological test results associated with psychiatric disorders in adults. *Psychological Bulletin, 85,* 141–162.

Hirsch, S.R., & Leff, J.P. (1971). Parental abnormalities of verbal communication in the transmission of schizophrenia. *Psychological Medicine, 1,* 118–127.

Hirsch, S.R., & Leff, J.P. (1975). *Abnormalities in parents of schizophrenics,* Maudsley monograph No. 22. London: Oxford University Press.

Howard, D., & Paterson, K.E. (1992). *The Pyramids and Palm Trees Test.* Bury St. Edmunds, UK: Thames Valley Test Co.

Humphreys, G.W., & Riddoch, M.J. (1987). *To see but not to see: A case study of visual agnosia.* Hove, UK: Lawrence Erlbaum Associates Ltd.

Kavanagh, D.J. (1992). Recent developments in expressed emotion and schizophrenia. *British Journal of Psychiatry, 160,* 601–620.

Kervetz, A. (1982). *Western Aphasia Battery.* San Antonio, CA: Psychological Corporation.

King, D.J. (1990). The effect of neuroleptics on cognitive and psychomotor function. *British Journal of Psychiatry, 157,* 799–811.

Kolb, B., & Whishaw, I.Q. (1983). Performance of schizophrenic patients on tests sensitive to left or right temporal or parietal function in neurological patients. *Journal of Nervous and Mental Disease, 171,* 435–443.

Kraepelin, E. (1913). *Dementia praecox and paraphrenia* [trans. R.M. Barclay, 1919]. Edinburgh: Livingstone.

Laws, K.R., Humber, S.A., Ramsey, D.J.C., & McCarthy, R.A. (1995a). Probing sensory and associative semantics for animals and objects in normal subjects. *Memory, 3,* 397–408.

Laws, K.R., McKenna, P.J., & McCarthy, R.A. (1995b). Delusions about people. *Neurocase, 1,* 349–362.

Lewis, S.W. (990). Computerised tomography in schizophrenia 15 years on. *British Journal of Psychiatry, 157,* supplement 9, 16–24.

Liddle, P.F., & Crow, T.J. (1984). Age disorientation in chronic schizophrenia is associated with global intellectual impairment. *British Journal of Psychiatry, 144,* 193–199.

Liddle, P.F., Friston, K.J., Frith, C.D., Hirsch, S.R., Jones, T., & Frackowiak, R.S.J. (1992). Patterns of cerebral blood flow in schizophrenia. *British Journal of Psychiatry, 60,* 179–186.

Liddle, P.F., & Morris, D.L. (1991). Schizophrenic symptoms and frontal lobe performance. *British Journal of Psychiatry, 158,* 340–345.

Malec, J. (1978). Neuropsychological assessment of schizophrenia versus brain damage: A review. *Journal of Nervous and Mental Disease, 166,* 507–516.

McKay, A.P., McKenna, P.J., Mortimer, A.M., Bentham, P., & Hodges, J.R. (1996). Semantic memory is impaired in schizophrenia. *Biological Psychiatry, 39,* 929–937.

McKenna, P., & Warrington, E.R. (1984). *The Graded Naming Test.* Windsor, UK: NFER-Nelson.

McKenna, P.J. (1994). *Schizophrenia and related syndromes.* Oxford: Oxford University Press.

McKenna, P.J., Clare, L., & Baddeley, A.D. (1995). Schizophrenia. In A.D. Baddeley, B.A. Wilson & F.N. Watts (Eds.), *Handbook of memory disorders.* Chichester, UK: Wiley.

McKenna, P.J., Tamlyn, D., Lund, C.E., Mortimer, A.M., Hammond, S., & Baddeley, A.D. (1990). Amnesic syndrome in schizophrenia. *Psychological Medicine, 20,* 967–972.

Morice, R. (1990). Cognitive inflexibility and pre-frontal dysfunction in schizophrenia and mania. *British Journal of Psychiatry, 157,* 50–54.

Nelson, H.E. (1976). A modified card sorting test sensitive to frontal lobe defects. *Cortex, 12,* 313–324.

Nelson, H.E. (1982). *The National Adult Reading Test (NART).* Windsor, UK: NFER-Nelson.

Osterrieth, P. (1944). Le test de copie d'une figure complexe. *Archives de Psychologie, 30,* 205–220.

Owens, D.G.C., & Johnstone, E.C. (1980). The disabilities of chronic schizophrenia—their nature and the factors contributing to their development. *British Journal of Psychiatry, 136,* 384–393.

Park, S., & Holzman, P.S. (1992). Schizophrenics show spatial working memory deficits. *Archives of General Psychiatry, 49,* 975–982.

Payne, R.W. (1973). Cognitive abnormalities. In H.J. Eysenck (Ed.), *Handbook of abnormal psychology.* London: Pitman.

Ron, M.A., & Harvey, I. (1990). The brain in schizophrenia. *Journal of Neurology, Neurosurgery and Psychiatry, 53,* 725–726.

Saykin, A.J., Gur, R.C., Gur, R.E., Mozley, P.D., Mozley, L.H., Resnick, S.M., Kester, D.B., & Stafiniak, P. (1991). Neuropsychological function in schizophrenia: Selective impairment in memory and learning. *Archives of General Psychiatry, 48,* 618–624.

Saykin, A.J., Shtasel, D.L., Gur, R.E., Kester, B., Mozley, L.H., Stafiniak, P., & Gur, R.C. (1994). Neuropsychological deficits in neuroleptic naive patients with first-episode schizophrenia. *Archives of General Psychiatry, 51,* 124–131.

Schuell, H.S., & Sefer, J.W. (1973). *Differential diagnosis of aphasia with the Minnesota Test, 2nd Edition, Revised.* Minneapolis: University of Minnesota Press.

Shallice, T., Burgess, P.W., & Frith, C.D. (1991). Can the neuropsychological case-study approach be applied to schizophrenia? *Psychological Medicine, 21,* 661–673.

Shallice, T., & Evans, M.E. (1978). The role of the frontal lobes in cognitive estimation. *Cortex, 14,* 294–303.

Snodgrass, J.G., & Vanderwart, M. (1980). A standardised set of 260 pictures: Norms for name agreement. *Journal of Experimental Psychology: General, 6,* 174–215.

Squire, L.R. (1987). *Memory and brain.* Oxford: Oxford University Press.

Stevens, M., Crow, T.J., Bowman, M.J., & Coles, E.C. (1978). Age disorientation in schizophrenia: A constant prevalence of 25 per cent in a chronic mental hospital population? *British Journal of Psychiatry, 133,* 130–136.

Stewart, F., Parkin, A.J., & Hunkin, N.M. (1992). Naming impairments following recovery from herpes simplex encephalitis: Category specific? *Quarterly Journal of Experimental Psychology, 44A,* 261–284.

Tamlyn, D., McKenna, P.J., Mortimer, A.M., Lund, C.E., Hammond, S., & Baddeley, A.D. (1992). Memory impairment in schizophrenia: Its extent, affiliations and neuropsychological character. *Psychological Medicine, 22,* 101–115.

Van Horn, J.D., & McManus, I.C. (1992). Ventricular enlargement in schizophrenia: A meta-analysis of studies of the ventricle:brain ratio (VBR). *British Journal of Psychiatry, 160,* 687–697.

Warrington, E.K., & James, M. (1991). *The Visual Object and Space Perception Battery.* Bury St Edmunds, UK: Thames Valley Test Company.

Warrington, E.K., & Taylor, A.M. (1973). The contribution of the right parietal lobe to object recognition. *Cortex, 9,* 152–164.

Wilson, B.A., Cockburn, J.M., & Baddeley, A.D. (1985). *The Rivermead Behavioural Memory Test.* Bury St. Edmunds, UK: Thames Valley Test Co.

9 Face Memory Impairment in the Cotard Delusion

Katharine M. Leafhead
*University of Durham, UK, MRC Applied Psychology Unit,
Cambridge, UK and UMDS, Division of Psychiatry and Psychology,
Guy's Hospital, London, UK*

Michael D. Kopelman
*UMDS, Academic Unit of Psychiatry, St. Thomas' Hospital,
London, UK*

INTRODUCTION

In 1882, Jules Cotard, a French psychiatrist, published a number of case reports in which the central feature was what he termed nihilistic delusions (*le délire de négation*). In their milder form, these delusions were characterised by self-deprecation and feelings of despair, and in their most extreme form by a total denial of the self and external world. The delusion was first referred to eponymously by Séglas following a suggestion by a contemporary, M. Régis (Séglas, 1897). Over the years, the term "Cotard syndrome" has become almost synonymous with the most striking feature found in the nihilistic delusions described by Cotard: the belief that one is dead. Cotard himself, however, believed that this symptom occurred in severe forms of *le délire de négation* and that it did not represent the defining feature. Consistent with Cotard's own view, Young and Leafhead (1996) recently argued that the term "syndrome" as applied to the Cotard delusion is at best unhelpful, not merely in terms of Cotard's original cases, but also in regard to other and more recent published cases; the term "syndrome" suggests the necessary co-occurrence of symptoms and this was not found for either set of case reports.

Until very recently, the Cotard delusion was either viewed in the psychiatric literature as just an intriguing curiosity (an "uncommon psychiatric syndrome") or it was interpreted in psychodynamic terms, for example, as a "death-wish inherent in the collective conscious" (Enoch &

165

Trethowan, 1979, p.130). Self-negation, self-punishment and feelings of guilt were all seen as reflections of this death-wish.

Over the past few years, however, an alternative theory of the Cotard delusion has been proposed (e.g. Young, Robertson, Hellawell, de Pauw, & Pentland, 1992). Young and his colleagues pointed to a number of perceptually anomalous experiences in the Cotard delusion. These anomalies involve things appearing unfamiliar and unreal to the patients, as well as a loss of emotional responsiveness. Indeed, as Young and Leafhead (1996) remark, Cotard himself noted the presence of perceptual abnormalities in his 1882 case reports; and they view their theory as an extension of Cotard's own view of the delusion. Furthermore, they have demonstrated the presence of impaired processing of faces and buildings in people who have suffered Cotard delusions (Wright, Young, & Hellawell, 1993; Young et al., 1992; Young, Leafhead, & Szulecka, 1994; Young & Leafhead, 1996). These findings followed investigation after an initial complaint by patient WI (Young et al., 1992) of a lack of feeling of familiarity for things that he saw: in particular, for buildings and people's faces. Formal testing revealed impairments in face processing, including recognition memory for faces and labelling of emotional facial expressions (Young et al., 1992). Similar patterns of impairment were found for patients KH (Wright et al., 1993) and JK (Young et al., 1994). In addition to complaining of a lack of feeling of familiarity for once-familiar things (i.e. buildings and people's faces), all three patients complained of feelings of unreality and feelings of derealisation and/or depersonalisation.

Young et al. (1992) noted that face-processing impairments are not in themselves sufficient to cause the Cotard delusion, as many brain-injured patients are impaired on tasks of face processing but do not believe they are dead. However, as Young and Leafhead (1996) noted, this does not mean that face processing impairments in the Cotard delusion are not significant. Rather, Young and his colleagues (Wright et al., 1993; Young et al., 1992) suggested that the failure to recognise once-familiar faces and buildings, and the underlying lack of feeling of familiarity for those things, may contribute to the onset and maintenance of the Cotard delusion by serving to heighten feelings of unreality. Hence, they argued that the Cotard delusion is the result of a misinterpretation of these anomalous perceptual experiences (Wright et al., 1993; Young et al., 1992; Young, 1994; Young et al., 1994; Young & Leafhead, 1996).

Leafhead, Young, and Szulecka (1996) noted that such experiences might potentially be interpreted in many possible ways and agreed with Kaney and Bentall's (1989) view that this will depend on social and personal factors. In regard to this, it is relevant that the Cotard delusion typically arises in the context of depression. Beck (1967, 1989) argued that depressed individuals commonly have a negative cognitive set, which consists of negative views of themselves, the external world, and the future. Central to this is the concept of memory schemas, consisting of previous negative events. These schemas become activated automatically whenever similar negative events are encountered, and they influence the way in which these new events are interpreted. Hence, the self, the situation, and the future are all perceived as being hopeless. The automaticity of schema activation leads the depressed individual to make inappropriate inferences about causation. For example, if the person to whom you are attracted does not feel the same attraction for you, it is because you are a fat, ugly, uninteresting failure—and you always will be.

Consistent with Beck's formulation of depression, it has been shown (e.g. Candido & Romney, 1990; Kaney & Bentall, 1989) that depressed individuals do indeed tend to attribute negative events to internal causes (*It's my fault*) rather than to external causes (*It's someone else's fault*). Drawing from this theory, Wright et al. (1993) suggested that the patients' depressed mood contributes to their seeking an internal cause for their perceptual problems, and concluding erroneously that they must be dead. That is to say, they (correctly) attribute their altered perceptual experience as being a change in themselves but (incorrectly) go on to infer that they are dead.

Young and Leafhead (1996) view this theory as an extension of Cotard's own conception of *le délire de négation*. Indeed, Cotard either made or anticipated a number of points that appear to have been forgotten in the research literature. It has already been mentioned that Cotard notes the presence of perceptual abnormalities. He also noted the presence of a loss of visual imagery (which frequently accompanies visual recognition impairments), and suggested that nihilistic delusions reflected a misinterpretation of this altered perception. Finally, and most importantly, Cotard's (1882, p.343) paper ends with a version of the attribution hypothesis in which he argues that in delusions of negation *"Le malade s'accuse lui-même"*. Young and his colleagues (e.g. Young & Leafhead, 1996) argue that this insight is central to understanding the Cotard delusion.

To summarise, Young and his colleagues have suggested that the Cotard delusion results from patients' attempts to explain perceptually anomalous experiences. These experiences include feelings that things seem unreal, a lack of feeling of familiarity for once-familiar faces and places, and a loss of emotional responsiveness. The patients' depressed mood leads them to seek an internal cause for these changes in perception, which in turn leads them to infer that they are dead.

In this chapter, we describe the case of a 61-year-old man who developed the Cotard delusion, and present evidence that is consistent with the theory held by Young and his colleagues.

CASE DESCRIPTION

RB is a 61-year-old man who became depressed and took an overdose following a bowel resection. He was transferred to a psychiatric ward of a general hospital, where he was initially prescribed fluoxetine, but it was soon realised that his depression was rather worse than first thought and his mood subsequently worsened. He began to say that he had been dead since the previous week. RB had no previous known psychiatric history, but his wife suffers from chronic schizophrenia and has done so for many years. RB had little formal education; he left school at the age of 14 with no qualifications, and he is only semi-literate.

RB believed that he was dead. He constantly looked at the ward clock and, when asked why, he said that he could not understand why the clock was still working; it should have stopped at the time he died. He became extremely anxious and frustrated at his inability to understand why the clock continued to move on in time. RB reported feeling as though he were not there, and at one time claimed to be "somewhere in between Heaven and Hell". Such feelings of unreality are consistent with previous reports of the Cotard delusion referred to earlier.

RB's behaviour was highly reminiscent of Cotard's (1882) description of patients suffering from *le délire de négation* who displayed "anxious agitation". He was extremely agitated and deeply distressed; he was unable to lie down or sit for very long and paced continually up and down at the side of his bed.

Testing was attempted on four occasions. On the first occasion, when he was convinced he was dead, RB was distressed, anxious, and extremely restless. We attempted to carry out some formal testing, but he became even more distressed and we decided to end the session after only a few minutes. We attempted to have a general conversation with him, but he had severe difficulty in concentrating. He returned to his bed space in an extremely anxious state, and paced up and down by the side of his bed for well over an hour.

A fortnight later, he was still disturbed and was able to complete one test only. After a further two weeks, testing was attempted again. In the intervening time, RB had been placed on a tricyclic anti-depressant and neuroleptic medication, had improved slightly, and was able to complete a number of tests. Although he was no longer fully convinced that he was dead, he still made occasional comments about the clock, and often looked up at it. Because he failed to respond to medication after a lengthy trial and remained distressed, ECT was resorted to, and his depression and delusional beliefs remitted rapidly.

About a week after ECT had been commenced, RB was seen again. During this session, RB spoke of having had several premonitions of events over the years, including of the deaths of his mother and his two brothers, and of his recent bowel operation. He reported being at work one day when, just after lunchtime, he had heard someone, whom he believed to be his mother, calling out his name. It later transpired that this was the time at which his mother had died. He further reported having sensed his mother the night before her funeral, when she was lying in an open coffin in his house. He said he was asleep and at first thought he was dreaming, but had "realised it was really her" when she touched him. Such phenomena are common in bereavement reactions (Parkes, 1972). He also said that she was present at his recent operation and had told him that "everything would be fine" and that he "would be alright", possibly indicative of the closeness of their relationship.

A year after his delusions remitted, RB underwent a closure of colostomy. He has not become deluded since, although he has been seen intermittently for episodes of depression. His wife remains very symptomatic.

FORMAL TESTING

Except where stated otherwise, the control data presented are those provided by Dr A. Young (see e.g. Young et al., 1995). The data were obtained from healthy controls (10 men, 10 women) with a mean age of 51.20 years (sd 6.06). They are not matched for IQ—we were unable to test IQ-matched controls, owing to the difficulty (see later) in measuring RB's pre-morbid and current IQ.

National Adult Reading Test (NART; Nelson, 1982)

The NART consists of 50 irregularly spelt words and provides an estimate of pre-morbid IQ. RB had an error score of 49, which gives an estimated pre-morbid full-scale IQ of 87. However, as stated, RB is only semi-literate, so little weight can be given to these scores, although they may be consistent with his low level of formal education. It is unfortunate that owing to the limited time during which RB could be tested, we were unable to measure his current level of IQ.

Benton word fluency (Benton, 1968)

RB was asked to name as many words (excluding proper nouns and names) as he could beginning with the letter "F". He was given one minute to do this. This was repeated with the letters and "A" and "S" respectively. He scored a total of 9 words (F=6; A=1; S=2). This is a very poor score—worse than many patients with severe dementia (Kopelman, 1991).

Middlesex Elderly Assessment of Mental State (Golding, 1989)

This is a test for screening gross impairment of specific cognitive skills in the elderly. We decided to test RB with this in an attempt to gain a clearer picture of RB's overall level of functioning, as well as to identify any particular areas of weakness. RB passed 8 of the 11 subtests, including orientation, comprehension, spatial construction, and motor preservation. In regard to memory, he passed the subtest concerned with remembering pictures. Of particular interest is that he passed the verbal fluency test, which is perhaps surprising, given his poor score on the Benton test (see previous paragraph), although it must be remembered that the test is designed to screen for *gross* impairment in the elderly. The tests he failed on were: name-learning, which involves learning the name of the photograph of a face; naming three objects (a watch, watch-strap, and watch-buckle); and, finally, arithmetic, which involves the addition or subtraction of three sets of two numbers (e.g. 6+4=?). This last result may again reflect RB's poor formal education.

Contrast Sensitivity

RB's contrast sensitivity function was tested using the Vistech 6000. It was found to be slightly below normal limits on the first testing session, but normal a fortnight later.

Warrington Recognition Memory Test (Warrington, 1984)

In the Warrington Recognition Memory Test (RMT), 50 faces are presented serially, each for three seconds. The subject is asked to make a judgement as to whether each face is pleasant or unpleasant (in order to facilitate encoding). Immediately following presentation of the series, each face is presented again, alongside a previously unseen distractor face in a forced-choice recognition task. The procedure for administering the words subtest is usually the same. However, as noted earlier, RB is only semi-literate. Hence, instead of his looking at the words, they were read out to him.

The results for the RMT (along with the tests described later) are presented in Table 9.1. RB was tested on three occasions: the first was when he believed he was dead; the second was when he was no longer fully convinced he was dead, but still highly disturbed and still making comments about, and looking at, the clock; and the third was after his delusion had remitted. The Table shows RB's raw scores for the numbers of faces and words he identified correctly, together with the percentile scores for age-matched controls. Also for the purposes of comparison, mean scores for a group of patients (n=134) with right hemisphere lesions, and a group (n=145) with left hemisphere lesions (reported by Warrington, 1984) are shown.

TABLE 9.1
Scores for RB with Control Age-matched Percentiles for the Warrington
Recognition Memory Test for Words and Faces

		FACES		WORDS	
		Accuracy (/50)	Percentile	Accuracy (/50)	Percentile
RB	Test 1	36	5th	39	25th
	Test 2	37	10th	41	25th
	Test 3	40	25th	not done	–
Right hemisphere lesions:					
		39.7		44.6	
Left hemisphere lesions:					
		41.8		39.9	

As the Table shows, RB scored only 36/50 for faces, and 39/50 for words. His score for faces was clearly worse than that for patients with right hemisphere lesions, while his score for words was in keeping with that for patients with left hemisphere lesions. The discrepancy between the faces and words subtests for RB (3) was small; although, as noted previously, it is difficult to gauge how much weight can be placed on RB's score for words, given his literacy problems. A problem arises as to the interpretation of these results in that the published mean score for faces for patients with right hemisphere lesions (mean=39.7, sd=6.7) falls within one standard deviation of that for normal controls in the 60–64 age group (mean=42.31, sd=4.37). The same is true for the mean score on the words subtest for patients with left hemisphere lesions (mean=39.9, sd=7.6) relative to that for age-matched controls (mean=43.22, sd=4.15). Given the problems of interpretation due to RB's semi-literacy, we conducted some more tests in order to obtain a clearer view of RB's visual recognition memory functioning.

Facial Identification

RB was shown the photographs of 20 faces, presented in random order. Half the faces were famous, rated for high familiarity (see Young et al., 1995). The other half consisted entirely of unfamiliar faces. RB was asked: (i) whether or not each face was familiar to him; (ii) whether he could state the occupation of the person shown; and (iii) whether he could name the person shown. The results are presented in Table 9.2.

As Table 9.2 shows, RB identified 19 of the 20 highly familiar faces as being familiar, was able to give the correct occupation for 16/20, but was able to name only 10 of them, which is lower than the mean of 16.10 for the

TABLE 9.2
RB's Performance on Face Processing Tasks Compared to Control Data

Facial identification	RB	Controls Mean	Sd
FACES: High-familiarity faces			
Familiarity	19/20	18.75	1.37
Occupation	16/20	18.50	1.67
Name	10/20	16.10	3.51
Correct rejections	20/20	18.70	1.42
NAMES: High-familiarity names			
Familiarity	18/20	not available	
Occupation	15/20	"	
Name	15/20	"	
Correct rejections	18/20	"	
Facial disguises test Total	21/24	22.30	2.16
Labelling of emotional facial expressions	18/24	21.10	1.70
Gaze direction	14/18	16.95	0.89
Recognition memory for unfamiliar buildings	37/50	43.35	2.25
Identification of famous buildings	13/20	15.30	3.85
Correct rejections	10/10	9.50	0.61

controls. He did not give any false positive; that is to say, he did not say that any of the unfamiliar faces were familiar to him. In the second part of the task, the names of all the faces (both famous and unfamiliar) previously shown were presented. RB was asked to identify the individuals from their names by: (i) stating whether the names were familiar to him; (ii) stating their occupations; and (iii) describing the appearance of the individuals. This part of the task is to ascertain whether RB knew who the people were in the cases in which he had been unable to identify them from their faces. There are no control data for this part of the task, but it is clear that RB was able to state the appearance of 15 of the faces, whereas he had only been able to name 10 of them from their faces. Finally, he made only two false positives, stating that two of the unfamiliar names were familiar to him.

Facial Disguises Test

In this test, the photographs of the faces of four people were presented to RB on a card. At the top of the card, each face sported some form of disguise (e.g. false moustache and spectacles). At the bottom of each card were the photographs of those people without disguises. RB was asked to identify which of each of the disguised faces corresponded to which of the individuals shown at the bottom of the card. There were two sets of stimuli. Table 9.2 shows RB's scores, together with those of 34 males aged 65–75 years (see Young, Ellis, Szulecka, & de Pauw, 1990a). RB's score was in keeping with those of the controls.

Labelling of Emotional Facial Expressions

RB was shown the photographs of 24 faces depicting a variety of emotional expressions, from the Ekman and Friesen (1976) series. Beneath each photograph was a list of six different emotional expressions; happiness, fear, disgust, sadness, surprise, and anger (see Young et al., 1990a). RB was asked to identify which label corresponded to the emotion shown on the face in each photograph. Table 9.2 shows RB's scores, together with those of the same controls reported on the disguises test (Young et al., 1990a). As Table 9.2 shows, RB scored 18/24, which is slightly lower than the mean control score of 21.1 (sd 1.7).

Gaze Direction

RB was presented with 18 pairs of photographs, always of the same male individual whose head was angled left, right, or straight ahead (see Young et al., 1995). In one of the pair, the face was looking directly ahead and in the other the eye gaze was either 5°, 10°, or 20° to the left or right. RB was asked to say in which face the eyes were looking directly towards him. As Table 9.2 shows, RB scored a total of 14/18, which is slightly lower than that of the controls. It is important to note, however, that all RB's errors were made on eye-gazes of 5° to the left or right: and these are more difficult to decide on than are those of 10° and 20°.

Recognition Memory for Buildings

In this task, the photographs of 50 unfamiliar buildings (houses) were presented serially for three seconds each (see Young et al., 1995). RB was asked to decide whether each building was pleasant or not (in order to facilitate encoding). Afterwards, the same buildings were shown again, but this time each was presented alongside a previously unseen distractor. RB was asked to identify which of each of the pairs of buildings he had been shown previously. He scored 37/50, which is lower than the controls' mean score (m = 43.35, sd = 2.25).

Identification of Famous Buildings

In this test (see Young et al., 1995), the photographs of 20 famous buildings (e.g. the Post Office Tower, the Parthenon, and the Sydney Opera House) were presented randomly, together with the photographs of 10 unfamiliar buildings, matched for similarity. RB was asked to say whether each building was familiar and, if it was, to provide its name. RB identified correctly 13 of the 20 buildings, and gave no false positives in terms of familiarity. His score was in keeping with that of the controls.

Magical Ideation Scale (MIS; Eckblad & Chapman, 1983)

In the MIS, 30 statements are presented to which the testee has to respond "true" or "false". Statements include: "I have had the momentary feeling that I might not be human" and "I think I could learn to read others' minds if I wanted to". Again owing to his fragile state, it was deemed best not to give this test to RB until the day of his discharge from hospital, after his delusions had remitted. Despite this, he scored 10, which is well above the control score of less than 3 (Eckblad & Chapman, 1983). It was during this test that he spoke of having had premonitions (noted earlier). Even though RB was no longer delusional, therefore, he still held some unusual beliefs. In particular, he agreed with the statements: "If reincarnation were true, it would explain some unusual experiences I have had" and "I have wondered whether the spirits of the dead can influence the living".

DISCUSSION

RB showed impaired recognition memory for words and faces (Warrington, 1984) and for buildings (Young et al., 1995), and also for the identification of faces (Young, de Haan, & Newcombe, 1990b). His performance on the labelling of emotional facial expressions test (Eckman & Friesen, 1976; Young et al., 1990b), however, was intact, as was his performance on the identification of buildings task, suggesting that his performance on face processing tasks was differentially affected. It is clear, however, that he did not show the pattern of impaired visual memory alongside intact verbal memory commonly seen in the Cotard delusion (e.g. Wright et al., 1993; Young et al., 1992; Young et al., 1994). As noted earlier, his impaired verbal processing is almost certainly explained by his being only semi-literate. There is no such explanation for his impaired visual memory.

Of particular interest is that the fact that while RB's recognition memory for faces and buildings, and his naming of famous faces, was impaired, his performance on the facial disguises and expression labelling tests was intact. This suggests that while RB's *memory* for faces was impaired, his ability to *process* faces in tasks requiring little or no memory function was unimpaired. This is consistent with Young and Leafhead's (1996) suggestion that the memory component of visual processing may be differentially affected in the Cotard delusion; all three patients in their report were impaired on tasks of visual processing, but especially so on memory for faces.

Young and his colleagues (Wright et al., 1993; Young et al., 1992; Young et al., 1994) have suggested a clear role for impaired memory for faces, places, and buildings, together with feelings of unreality and unfamiliarity, in the formation of the Cotard delusion. The presence of face processing deficits in RB, together with his reported feelings of unreality, lend support to Young's theory. As noted earlier, however, it is important to note that Young et al. (1992) and Wright et al. (1993) do not suggest visual processing deficits and feelings of unreality are in themselves sufficient cause for the Cotard delusion to emerge; such things are experienced by many people who do not conclude that they are dead. The key interaction is between face processing deficits, feelings of unreality, and depression. As noted earlier, Wright et al. (1993) suggested that depression leads patients to seek an internal cause for their altered perceptual experience. Although the attribution of these changes is correctly internalised, the consequences of them are exaggerated. This, in turn, leads patients to conclude erroneously that they must be dead. This hypothesis fits neatly with the case of RB.

Of additional interest is RB's perception of time as indicated by his pre-occupation with the clock; time, according to RB, should have stopped because he was dead. This in itself is noteworthy, as most of us are aware that time continues after we are dead. Of particular interest, however, is the fact that the Cotard delusion is associated with frontal (as well as right temporo-parietal) lobe damage (e.g. Drake, 1988; Joseph & O'Leary, 1986; Young et al., 1992). Frontal lobe damage has been associated with impaired memory for temporal context (e.g. Mayes, Meudell, & Pickering, 1985; Shimamura et al., 1990), although there are two other views concerning temporal context deficits in organic amnesia. The first is that temporal context memory impairment is the result of diencephalic amnesia (e.g. Parkin, Leng, & Hunkin, 1990), while the second suggests that the temporal context memory deficit forms part of the primary amnesic disorder (e.g. Huppert & Piercy, 1978; Kopelman, 1989, 1991). Parenthetically, Ornstein (1975, p.93) noted that "Clock time is an important element in the active mode of consciousness." That a disturbance in the appreciation of the linear progression of time was displayed by a patient suffering from the Cotard delusion underscores this notion.

In conclusion, rather than attempting to find "*the* cause of the Cotard delusion" (Young & Leafhead, 1996, p.166), Young and his colleagues (Young et al., 1992; Wright et al., 1993) have identified the roles of a number of contributory factors, and specified the interactions between them. RB's Cotard delusion arose in the context of depression, and he displayed impaired memory for faces and buildings, and complained about feelings of unreality. Such a pattern is consistent with the view that the face processing impairments seen in patients suffering from the Cotard delusion may heighten feelings of unreality and so contribute to the onset and maintenance of that delusion.

ACKNOWLEDGEMENTS

This work was made possible through an MRC Research Studentship to KML (under the supervision of Dr A. Young) and a grant from the Special Trustees of St. Thomas' Hospital (KML, MDK). We thank Dr A. Young for providing us with control data.

REFERENCES

Beck, A.T. (1967). *Depression: Clinical, experimental, and theoretical aspects*. New York: Harper & Row.

Beck, A.T. (1989). *Cognitive therapy and the emotional disorders*. Harmondsworth, UK: Penguin.

Benton, A.L. (1968). Differential behavioral effects of frontal lobe disease. *Neuropsychologia*, *6*, 53–60.

Candido, C.L., & Romney, D.M. (1990). Attributional style in paranoid vs. depressed patients. *British Journal of Medical Psychology*, *63*, 355–363.

Cotard, J. (1882). Du délire de négation. *Archives de Neurologie*, *4*, 152–170, 282–295.

Drake, M.E.J. (1988). Cotard's syndrome and temporal lobe epilepsy. *Psychiatric Journal of the University of Ottawa*. *13*, 36–39.

Eckblad, M., & Chapman, L.J. (1983). Magical ideation as an indicator of schizotypy. *Journal of Consulting and Clinical Psychology*, *51*, 215–225.

Ekman, P., & Friesen, W. (1976). *Pictures of facial affect*. Palo Alto, CA: Consulting Psychologists Press.

Enoch, M.D., & Trethowan, W.H. (1979). *Uncommon psychiatric syndromes* (2nd Edn.). Bristol: Wright & Sons.

Golding, E. (1989). *The Middlesex Elderly Assessment of Mental State*. Bury St. Edmunds, UK: Thames Valley Test Company.

Joseph, A.B., & O'Leary, D.H. (1986). Brain atrophy and interhemispheric fissure enlargement in Cotard's syndrome. *Journal of Clinical Psychiatry*, *47*, 518–520.

Kaney, S., & Bentall, R.P. (1989). Persecutory delusions and attributional style. *British Journal of Medical Psychology*, *62*, 191–198.

Huppert, F.A., & Piercy, M. (1978). The role of trace strength in recency and frequency judgements by amnesic and control subjects. *Quarterly Journal of Experimental Psychology*, *30*, 347–354.

Kopelman, M.D. (1989). Remote and autobiographical memory, temporal context memory and frontal atrophy in Korsakoff and Alzheimer patients. *Neuropsychologia*, *27*, 436–460.

Kopelman, M.D. (1991). Frontal lobe dysfunction and memory deficits in the alcoholic Korsakoff syndrome and Alzheimer-type dementia. *Brain*, *114*, 117–137.

Leafhead, K.M., Young, A.W., & Szulecka, T.K. (1996). Delusions demand attention. *Cognitive Neuropsychiatry*, *1*, 5–16.

Mayes, A.R., Meudell, P.R., & Pickering, A. (1985). Is organic amnesia caused by a selective deficit in remembering contextual information? *Cortex, 21*, 167–202.

Nelson, H.E. (1982). *The National Adult Reading Test (NART): Test Manual.* Windsor, UK: NFER-Nelson.

Ornstein, R.E. (1975). *The psychology of consciousness.* Harmondsworth, UK: Penguin Books Limited.

Parkes, C.M. (1972). *Bereavement: Studies of grief in adult life.* London: Tavistock Press.

Parkin, A.J., Leng, N.R.C., & Hunkin, N. (1990). Differential sensitivity to contextual information in diencephalic and temporal lobe amnesia. *Cortex, 26*, 373–380.

Séglas, J. (1897). *Le délire des négations: Séméiologie et diagnostic.* Paris: Masson, Gauthier-Villars.

Shimamura, A.P., Janowsky, J.S., & Squire, L.R. (1990). Memory for the order of events in patients with frontal lobe lesions and amnesic patients. *Neuropsychologia, 28*, 803–813.

Warrington, E.K. (1984). *Recognition Memory Test.* Windsor, UK: NFER-Nelson.

Wright, S., Young, A.W., & Hellawell, D.J. (1993). Sequential Cotard and Capgras delusions. *British Journal of Clinical Psychology, 32*, 345–349.

Young, A.W., Aggleton, J.P., Hellawell, D.J., Johnson, M., Broks, P., & Hanley, J.R. (1995). Face processing impairments after amygdalotomy. *Brain, 118*, 15–24.

Young, A.W., de Haan, E.H.F., & Newcombe, F. (1990b). Unawareness of impaired face recognition. *Brain and Cognition, 14*, 1–18.

Young, A.W., Ellis, H.D., Szulecka, T.K., & de Pauw, K.W. (1990a). Face processing impairments and delusional misidentification. *Behavioural Neurology, 3*, 153–168.

Young, A.W., & Leafhead, K.M. (1996). Betwixt life and death: Case studies of the Cotard delusion. In P.W. Halligan & J.C. Marshall (Eds.), *Method in madness: Case studies in cognitive neuropsychiatry.* Hove, UK: Psychology Press.

Young, A.W., Leafhead, K.M., & Szulecka, T.K. (1994). The Capgras and Cotard delusion. *Psychopathology, 27*, 226–231.

Young, A.W., Robertson, I.H., Hellawell, D.J., de Pauw, K.W., & Pentland, B. (1992). Cotard delusion after brain injury. *Psychological Medicine, 22*, 799–804.

10

Coping with Amnesia: The Natural History of a Compensatory Memory System

Barbara A. Wilson
MRC Applied Psychology Unit, Cambridge, UK

JC, and Evie Hughes
London, UK

INTRODUCTION

As disorders of memory are common in subjects who have experienced brain injury through a variety of reasons, therapists and those affected by such injury have employed several strategies in attempts to alleviate or compensate for memory loss. Among these strategies, external memory aids are probably the most effective in the long run, and therefore the most likely to be used (Wilson, 1991). However, external aids are often difficult for memory-impaired people to use efficiently because remembering to employ an aid is in itself a memory task. Thus the very people who need external memory aids most are those who have the greatest difficulty in learning to use them. Despite this somewhat daunting barrier it would seem essential to aim for compensation of memory employing a potentially effective means such as external aids, given that *restoration* of memory functioning following organic amnesia would appear to be an unrealistic alternative goal.

Note: An earlier version of this chapter appeared in *Neuropsychological Rehabilitation*, 1997, 7, 43–56.

Evidence that at least some memory-impaired people can learn to compensate effectively was found in a long-term follow-up study of people referred for memory therapy several years earlier, when Wilson (1991) found that most of her subjects had in the intervening years learned coping methods for bypassing or compensating their memory problems by using external aids and strategies. Kime, Lamb, and Wilson (1996) report the case of a young woman who exhibited dense amnesia following status epilepticus. With intensive therapy and a comprehensive programme of cueing by staff at a rehabilitation centre, the young woman learned to use a number of external aids very efficiently. In addition, the subject demonstrated generalisation of this compensatory behaviour by employing the aids in new environments and for new problems. The programme was successful enough to enable the subject to return to paid employment.

Wilson and Watson (1996) consider some of the factors that predict successful use of compensatory strategies in people with non-progressive memory impairment. They suggest that age, absence of additional cognitive deficits (that is a pure amnesic syndrome), and a screening score of at least 3 of a possible 12 points on the Rivermead Behavioural Memory Test (Wilson, Cockburn, & Baddeley, 1985) are all good predictors of (a) independence and (b) using at least six memory aids or strategies in daily living. One of the subjects in the Wilson (1991) study, and also described briefly in Wilson (1995), is JC, a young man who makes extremely good use of external aids and compensatory strategies. Despite a severe amnesia, JC lives alone and is self-employed. Because of JC's success and because he is constantly refining and developing his compensatory system, we present here a natural history of its development to date, in the belief that this history will throw light on the processes involved in enabling people with amnesia to develop efficient ways of coping with their memory problems.

CASE HISTORY

JC was born in 1965. At school he obtained a scholarship to study law at Cambridge University. During his second year at university, at the age of 20, he sustained an epileptic seizure and collapsed during a tutorial. He was admitted to the accident and emergency department of the local hospital where he had two further seizures. A CT scan, carried out soon after, showed a large sub-arachnoid haemorrhage arising from the left occipital region. A subsequent arteriogram showed a left posterior cerebral artery aneurysm. The aneurysm was clipped three weeks later.

About five weeks after the haemorrhage, JC was admitted to a rehabilitation unit for a further five weeks' treatment. On admission to rehabilitation, JC was reported as having a marked loss of memory and not being able to remember anything from one minute to the next. His "higher functions" seemed intact and there was no dysphasia. Neurological examination revealed a dense right hemianopia with macular sparing and diplopia, and some meningeal irritation.

When discharged from rehabilitation, JC's diplopia had resolved although he still had the hemianopia. He remained with a severe memory impairment and was referred to one of the present authors (BAW) for advice on the management of his memory difficulties. He was seen approximately once every two weeks between June and December 1986 for memory assessment and advice. However, much of JC's rehabilitation treatment was conducted independently by JC himself and his family.

Following a brief description of the neuropsychological assessment and initial treatment approaches, this paper will focus on the development of JC's own coping strategies from accounts provided by JC and his aunt, Evie Hughes.

NEUROPSYCHOLOGICAL ASSESSMENT

JC was assessed on tests of general intellectual functioning, naming, memory, perception, executive skills, and reading. His general intellectual functioning was in the superior range of ability; his scores on all tests of naming, visuospatial and visuoperceptual functioning, reading, and executive skills were all above average. It was only on tests of memory that JC's scores gave cause for concern. On the RBMT his screening score was 1 out of a maximum of 12. Most normal control subjects score at least 10 out of 12 and a score of 3 or less is in the severely impaired range.

On the Wechsler Memory Scale–Revised (Wechsler, 1987) JC scored in the average range for tests involving immediate memory and in the severely impaired range for delayed recall. He had no difficulty with attention and concentration. On the Recognition Memory Test (Warrington, 1984) JC scored at chance level, that is once again in the severely impaired range. On tests of retrograde amnesia his scores were normal except for events that had happened since his haemorrhage. He was able to recall events shortly before his haemorrhage, including being at the tutorial where he collapsed. Thus any retrograde amnesia appeared to have resolved. JC had all the characteristics of a pure amnesic syndrome: his immediate memory was good, he had problems after a delay or distraction; he had difficulty learning new information and his cognitive skills (other than memory) were intact.

EARLY REHABILITATION

With regard to the treatment strategies investigated during June to December 1986, we concentrated on (a) external aids, (b) mnemonics, (c) rehearsal strategies, and (d) chaining. A summary of the treatment report of December 1986 follows:

(a) *External aids*: J uses his diary and notebook efficiently although he is likely to write the same thing twice. I gave him some information about the Casio databank wrist-watch and I understand his father is going to get one on approval.

(b) *Mnemonics*: J is able to benefit from first-letter mnemonics and from the face–name visual imagery procedure in an experimental setting. He claims to use the face–name method to help remember people when he is serving in his father's shop. I am sure the mnemonics are of limited value in everyday life but if he needs to learn certain limited pieces of information, mnemonics may well help.

(c) *Rehearsal*: I compared J's ability to recall verbal material using (i) the PQRST method [Preview, Question, Read, State, and Test, Robinson, 1970] and (ii) Rote rehearsal. He was able to learn some material with both methods. Neither was superior to the other. It would be worth investigating the method of expanding rehearsal (Landauer & Bjork, 1978).

(d) *Chaining*, i.e. breaking a task down into steps and teaching one step at a time: This method was used successfully to teach J short routes.

Conclusion

The conclusions to the 1986 report were as follows:

J still has considerable memory problems although he retains some information reasonably well. For example, he gave a good and fairly detailed account of a recent trip to the USA but he repeated segments of the account during the same conversation and gave me the same account twice more during the same session. He still shows evidence of everyday memory difficulties. For example, he learned where my room was during July. In August I moved to another room further along the same corridor but J has never learned the way to this room and still waits outside the original room.

Obviously it is going to be enormously difficult for him to resume his studies. I am not sure if J and his father are aware of how handicapping his problems are. I have spoken to Mr. C (senior) on several occasions but I am not sure whether he is ready to be told that J is extremely unlikely to complete his degree. One of my difficulties is that I do not know what message the neurosurgeon has given the family. Perhaps the rather gloomy outlook should be broached by the neurosurgeon? Anyway, I am sending him a copy of this letter and leave it in the hands of the Cambridge team to advise. I am willing to contact the family again if you think this is best.

In addition to his visits to BAW, JC, Evie Hughes and other family members became involved in developing a compensatory system to enable JC to live as independently as possible. At the time of writing this process has been in operation for 10 years. Even today modifications continue. A summary of the development of this system follows. JC's account of this development is presented next, with Evie's account following.

JC's System (From his Notes)

Stage 1: Between October and December 1986, I used a notebook which I kept in my shirt pocket and a watch with an alarm which sounded every hour. Whenever the alarm sounded, I noted down what I was doing. Later I transferred this information to a journal but I did little in the way of forward planning.

Stage 2: "The Grand Plan" January 1987. I had a weekly sheet on my desk and a daily sheet which I filled in with details from my weekly sheet and one-off appointments from my diary. The daily card was kept in a small diary. The proposal was:

1. *All* appointments were to be written down.
2. There would be a daily card in my diary.
3. A written list would be on my desk of all daily and weekly tasks (the weekly sheet).
4. Tasks would be transferred to my daily card in the evening or the morning. Evie, or one of my sisters would prompt me to do this.

Initially I used the back of my appointments diary as a record of the day. Very soon however, I used a spiral bound notebook instead. The diary was strapped with an elastic band to the notebook, and both fitted into the top pocket of my shirt. At this stage it was important that I carried the notebook on my person at all times.

The emphasis was now on forward planning and not concentrating on the past.

Stage 3: I obtained a dictaphone to record ongoing events which I transcribed into my journal in the evening.

Stage 4: April 1987. When writing the daily card I used the pocket diary as well as the weekly sheet. This was an attempt to set up a routine whereby when the alarm goes for an appointment, it is reset for the next appointment on the daily card. (This was never very successful, even at the time of getting my Seiko RC 4000 watch in 1989.)

Stage 5: In September 1987 I moved to my own flat in the same road as my parents' home. I removed the old front door key from my key ring so I would not go there by mistake.

Stage 6: October 1987. There was a problem of how I was to get information out of the diary since, as I read through it, I would forget what I was looking for. One of my sisters gave me a small loose-leaf diary, similar to a thin filofax, which seemed to help.

Stage 7: December 1987. I missed appointments because of forgetting to set my watch, so I made an extra effort to do this.

Stage 8: January 1988. I bought a filofax.

Stage 9: February 1988. In early February I missed an appointment with my youngest sister. She got cross with me to see if this would help. It seemed to have worked as I kept three extraordinary appointments during the week.

Stage 10: March 1988. My watch setting was better.

Stage 11: April 1988. Watch setting OK now. I was making notes in my filofax of the time spent on my projects.

Stage 12: July 1988. I started typing to see if a computer would be useful. I worked out the framework of a computer programme which would help me retrieve information from my diary.

Stage 13: September 1988. I started at the London College of Furniture. I had maps showing me how to get there as well as a note to get on the front of the train so I used the right exit of the station.

Stage 14: 13 October 1988. I looked into the possibility of using a computer for recording my diary. There were problems of the size of the database and also problems getting information out of the database.

Practical skills were developed without me being aware of how this came about. I could do things without being able to explain how.

Stage 15: February 1989. My diary was typed on to the computer. I was given a new watch, a Seiko RC 4000. Instructions for putting information into the watch were written on a sheet in my filofax. Six weeks later I had memorised these stages.

Stage 16: April 1989. When away from home I used my coat as a base. I used my dictaphone to plan my course work and found it was best to do the planning at the end of each lesson.

My college binder had different sections for different skills. For shopping I now had different sections for different shops rather than putting everything on one list. So, for example, groceries would go in one section and meat in another.

Stage 17: September 1990. I started courses at the Twickenham and Richmond College. I used an A–Z map on the bus to know when to get off. After 20 journeys, I knew without checking the map, when to get off. I had a map of the college grounds to get to the workshop and another map to get from Twickenham to Richmond. Finally I had notes on bus numbers and the position of the stops.

Stage 18 (since 1990): In January 1991 I had a date with a girl friend. The notes I made on my dictaphone during the evening were put on to a yellow sheet, with her name at the top, in my filofax. Later I called this a social sheet. Notes from later meetings were added to go on the sheet. A second and third sheet followed. I then used social sheets for other people. A colleague at work holds the record and he currently has nine social sheets. Most of these will be stored in a reserve file. Sticky back "post it" notes are put on to the social sheets with suggestions and ideas for future joint activities, when to make the next telephone call and so forth. Gradually different coloured sheets were used for different aspects of my life.

Whenever anything had to be done to my flat a green sheet was used. The pilot light on my boiler periodically gets clogged so I need to call in the plumber. He is currently on his third social sheet. Details of what needs to be done are written on "post it" notes so I know what to say when I phone him. Once the work has been done I enter it on the social sheet.

If I come across a restaurant I particularly like I note this on a red sheet. I include the name, the phone number, the address, how to get there, the kind of food served and some idea of how much a meal would cost. I then make a note of when I've been and with whom, and how much I spent. I occasionally note a particular good dish, e.g. "Beef with sweet basil is fab."

I began to use pink sheets in March 1995 for miscellaneous information such as notes on a new swimming pool that had opened nearby, or details of a holiday which required coordination of various dates or train times. I now call these "leisure sheets". The final kind of sheet is blue and I will say more about this in the next section.

Stage 19: Since 1992 I have been self-employed. I French polish and re-cane and re-rush chairs. The current system is this: A customer will phone and say he has a job for me. If it is to re-cane or re-rush a chair, the chair is usually delivered to me but sometimes I will collect it. If it is a French polishing job I need to go out to provide a quote.

I then open a job sheet in my filofax. A job number goes on the sheet together with the client's name, address and telephone number. I also record the date the job began, the deadline for completion, the type of job, the price quoted and job details. The job number corresponds with a numbered page in an A5 duplicate book. This process is slightly modified for work with dealers.

I take the customer's details and we agree a time when I will provide a quote. I make a note on the relevant daily sheet "To job 455". I also set my watch alarm so I leave in good time. I quote for the job and the customer retains the top copy from the job book as a record of what has been agreed. We also agree a time when I will return (or when the customer will collect). I note on my daily sheet in the filofax when I will carry out the job and also set the watch alarm. I note how long I spend on each job and log this in the job book and on the job sheet. I also note the cost of materials. When the customer pays, this is recorded in the job book, and the job sheet in the filofax is discarded.

I often take on work for dealers and other business firms. These are likely to lead to repeat orders. I record the dealer's details as with individual clients, but also note when I introduced myself to the dealer. The dealers' sheets are blue.

These coloured sheets and their cross-referencing capability give a capacity to retrieve information which is of more value than a computer program because several sheets can be viewed at the same time. It is also more portable and less prone to theft. The fact that the sheets are different colours makes them easier to find in my filofax.

Evie's Account

In the beginning I saw J every day, then three times a week. When he went to college, I saw him twice a week and by 1991 this had dropped to once a week. I was known as "a mobile resource unit", I filtered things out for him. Now he only comes when something important crops up like dealing with bureaucratic difficulties. For the last three years J has been self-sufficient. He still needs to have regular breaks for his meals and if he doesn't eat he gets ratty. If he is going out to dinner he may decide to eat a snack before he goes in case the meal is delayed.

J has a comprehensive system of memory aids, some of which have been modified to suit his particular needs. In his filofax he has a page a day diary which replaced his daily sheet. He also has extra pages which he can substitute for the originals in case errors are made or there are changes of plan. He flags up important messages, particularly changes of routine, by using sticky back "post it" notes. He crosses off tasks when they are completed. He has a map of the local area and uses coloured sheets for friends and activities. Every person in his life has a sheet with relevant information on.

Some lists are kept in his filofax. J uses six different kinds of lists. First there are the shopping lists. He writes on the list as things start running out. He also writes on the lists things he is likely to need when he plans his menus. He checks his cupboard to see if there is anything he should add and cheques are attached to his shopping list to act as a reminder to go to the bank or post office.

He also makes lists of telephone calls. All calls are logged to make sure they are not duplicated. There is a note in the filofax to make the due call which is also entered on to the watch alarm. Once it has been made, this note is ticked so he knows he has done it. The details of the call are entered into social or client sheets and also on to the dictaphone.

The third kind of list is for his accounts. He records all money coming in and going out, and therefore can quickly check whether he has done something.

Fourth is the menu chart which is planned every few weeks for the meals he eats alone or with friends. This ensures he does not eat the same things too often and that he has a balanced diet with seasonal foods. He also cross references these menus with his filofax, noting when he will be eating out and when friends will be coming over.

The fifth kind of list is for packing. These cover packing for going away and packing tools to take out with him. As J is self-employed and restores furniture he needs to keep a detailed account of his work so the final kind of list is his business account and job list. The progress of each job and the time taken is logged.

The lists are all kept in the appropriate place. For example, the menu chart is in the kitchen and the telephone list is by the phone.

The watch J uses now is a Seiko RC 4000, which was produced in small batches and is no longer made. This has several functions including (a) repeat weekly alarms—up to 15 of these can be programmed, each consisting of 12 letters; (b) one-off alarms—again a maximum of 15 of these can be entered with a maximum of 12 letters per message; (c) data sheets, of which there are 30, but J hardly ever uses them. The weekly alarms are used for classes, e.g. an upholstery class, swimming, and circuit training, and also for watering his plants and other regularly occurring tasks.

The one-off alarms are used for individual events and short-term reminders. So, for example, J enters an appointment in his watch system alarm (this is also entered into his filofax) and he also enters reminders such as "check the cooking" or "clean contact lenses". J now sets the watch automatically but has difficulty if this process is interrupted.

J has used other practical aids in the past. When he moved to his own flat he removed the previous flat's key from his key ring. He also role-played difficult situations to help reduce the emotions that got in the way of social encounters. When he used to serve in a shop he would repeat to himself, "I'm serving Mrs Big Nose" or whatever was appropriate whenever he had to leave the customer to find something.

He used to go rowing and take part in races. When he arrived, instead of waiting around he would change and do some exercises so he did not get bored and leave early. When the details of the racing starts were decided J wrote these on a piece of paper and stuck it in his sock. Once in the boat he saw the note and transferred it to a convenient crack at his feet to remind him which procedure had been chosen.

There are other strategies which J still uses. When leaving his seat on a plane or train he repeats continuously something like, "Third row on the left" or whatever. In his flat he always keeps everything in the same place and returns things to their appropriate place after use. He uses sticky backed "post-it" notes regularly to remind him to "make lunch" or that he has "made lunch". These notes are kept on a cupboard door in the kitchen.

An important aid, which is taken so much for granted that I nearly forgot to include it, is J's pocket dictaphone. He uses this during the day to record messages to himself. These can be about whom he meets, what he does, or what he needs to do. In the evening he transcribes the tape and makes the appropriate entry in his filofax or sets his watch alarm for future action. The dictaphone may be a back-up system to the appointment diary or it may be complementary to it. This may be illustrated by the following example at the time when J was applying for a second year at college.

1. Evie asked J about the application.
2. J made a note on the dictaphone.
3. In the evening J listened to the tape and wrote a note in his filofax about asking for the form and set the watch alarm to remind him to look in the filofax at a suitable time when he was in college.
4. When the alarm goes off J is reminded to look in his filofax and speak to his tutor.
5. J records on the dictaphone the tutor's response, goes immediately to fetch the form and makes a note on the dictaphone.
6. In the evening J puts papers ready to take to his regular meeting with Evie.
7. J discusses the form and fills it in.
8. The completed form is photocopied and a note made on the dictaphone.
9. In the evening one copy is filed and the other put with his college work and the watch is set to remind him to hand in the form.

Finally, J follows certain routines to avoid errors. The steps in his getting up and winding down routines are always carried out in the same order and in a social setting he will firmly ask for space to process information immediately before he forgets.

DISCUSSION

When asked about his system JC once said "I try to make the system foolproof. It's like a web, it's hard for anything to slip through the system. If I miss it with one thing I'll pick it up with another. I've individualised the system. It's constantly developing and I'm constantly refining and correcting it." Although it is unlikely that JC's system is absolutely foolproof, there is no doubt that he has developed an extremely effective compensatory structure that enables him to live independently and earn his own living. This is not easy for someone with such severe memory impairments. We must ask ourselves why it is that JC has succeeded when others have failed. The predictions made by Wilson and Watson (1996) are borne out to some extent. They found that people younger than 30 years of age at the time of insult were more likely to be independent, and indeed JC was 20 years old at the time of his haemorrhage. Wilson and Watson also found that memory-impaired people without additional cognitive deficits were more likely to compensate adequately and to be more independent than those with more widespread problems. JC has a pure amnesic syndrome.

Although Wilson and Watson noted that people obtaining at least 3 screening score points on the RBMT were more likely to compensate and be independent than those scoring 2 or less, this was not true for JC who scored only 1 on the test each time he was tested. A possible explanation for this discrepancy, and indeed an explanation for his exceptional success in the long term, lies in the outstanding intelligence shown by JC. His frontal lobes were not affected at all by the haemorrhage and, by his own account, he was always extremely well organised, even as a small child. Thus the combination of youth, intelligence, organised behaviour, determination, lack of additional cognitive deficits, and of course a fully supportive and imaginative family who worked with him at every stage of his problems, goes a long way in explaining JC's achievement of independence both in work and at home despite the severity of his memory impairment. He also had several months of rehabilitation, first as an in-patient and later as an out-patient, and although the effect of this cannot be measured there is some evidence to suggest that people receiving rehabilitation do better in the long run than those who do not receive it (Brooks, 1991; Cope, Cole, Hall, & Barkan, 1991; Greenwood & McMillan, 1993; McMillan & Greenwood, 1993).

An interesting comment made by JC in his account of the development of his system was that he learned practical skills without knowing how he had learned them. In common with other amnesic people, JC's implicit memory appeared normal and he was undoubtedly using this intact memory system when learning some of the skills he demonstrated in his daily routine. Evie notes that he learned to type without consciously being aware of how he achieved this skill, and this is a good example of procedural or implicit learning. The fact that JC successfully completed a course at a furniture college is probably due in part to the fact that he was able to bring his implicit memory into play. JC himself feels that his ability to learn practical skills was a big advantage. He also said that he considered it a big step forward when he started to do things twice as this proved "the system was beginning to work". He then had to refine procedures to prevent himself repeating things. The system is still not perfect and he finds, for example, that he telephones people twice with the same information. Nevertheless, JC has achieved an impressive level of independence in the face of a severe amnesic syndrome.

While most other memory-impaired people may be less intelligent than JC, and less fortunate in that most are likely to suffer more general damage involving cognitive skills other than memory, JC's success shows what can be achieved by patience, ingenuity, and commitment, as exhibited by himself and other members of his family; and although the degree of sophistication reached by JC in his use of compensatory memory aids may be beyond the level likely to be achieved by less gifted individuals, his efforts can at least be emulated in treatment programmes that of necessity will require more intensive rehabilitation and support along the way.

REFERENCES

Brooks, D.N. (1991). The effectiveness of post-acute rehabilitation. *Brain Injury*, *5*, 102–149.

Cope, D.N., Cole, J.R., Hall, K.M., & Barkan, H. (1991). Brain injury: Analysis of outcome in a post-acute rehabilitation system. *Brain Injury*, *5*, 111–139.

Greenwood, R.J., & McMillan, T.M. (1993). Models of rehabilitation programmes for the brain-injured adult I: Current provision, efficacy and good practice. *Clinical Rehabilitation*, *7*, 248–255.

Kime, S.K., Lamb, D.G., & Wilson, B.A. (1996). Use of a comprehensive program of external cuing to enhance procedural memory in a patient with dense amnesia. *Brain Injury*, *10*, 17–25.

Landauer, T.K., & Bjork, R.A. (1978). Optimum rehearsal patterns and name learning. In M.M. Gruneberg, P.E. Morris, & R.N. Sykes (Eds.), *Practical aspects of memory* (pp. 625–632). London: Academic Press.

McMillan, T.M., & Greenwood, R.J. (1993). Model of rehabilitation programmes for the brain-injured adult II: Model services and suggestions for change in the UK. *Clinical Rehabilitation*, *7*, 346–355.

Robinson, F.P. (1970). *Effective study*. New York: Harper & Row.

Warrington, E.K. (1984). *The Recognition Memory Test*. Windsor, UK: NFER-Nelson.

Wechsler, D. (1987). *The Wechsler Memory Scale–Revised*. San Antonio, CA: The Psychological Corporation.

Wilson, B.A. (1991). Long term prognosis of patients with severe memory disorders. *Neuropsychological Rehabilitation*, *1*, 117–134.

Wilson, B. A. (1995). Management and remediation of memory problems in brain-injured adults. In A.D. Baddeley, B.A. Wilson, & F.N. Watts (Eds.), *Handbook of memory disorders* (pp. 451–479). Chichester, UK: John Wiley.

Wilson, B.A., Cockburn, J., & Baddeley, A.D. (1985). *The Rivermead Behavioural Memory Test*. Bury St. Edmunds, UK: Thames Valley Test Company.

Wilson, B.A., & Watson, P.C. (1996). A practical framework for understanding compensatory behaviour in people with organic memory impairment. *Memory*, *4*, 465–486.

11 Take Note: Using Errorless Learning to Promote Memory Notebook Training

Ella J. Squires
University of Sussex, UK

Nicola M. Hunkin
University of Sheffield, UK

Alan J. Parkin
University of Sussex, UK

INTRODUCTION

One of the most common outcomes of brain injury is a memory impairment, manifest in an inability to remember new information. This anterograde deficit is often the greatest barrier to effective rehabilitation and can result in behaviour that is difficult for carers to cope with. Repetitive questioning is one of the most frequently reported behavioural problems faced by those who care for people with acquired memory impairments. The inability to remember new information forces memory-disordered people to rely on their carers for day-to-day information which, once provided, is usually not retained, resulting in persistent requests for the same information.

In this chapter we describe a study involving a 70-year-old stroke victim, Mr S, who presented with a dense anterograde amnesia. A major problem reported by his wife, Mrs S, was persistent repetitive questioning about the events of the day, such as what was for dinner and what time were they going out. Mr S had become wholly reliant on his wife for information and Mrs S admitted to feelings of exasperation at Mr S's frequent questioning. The aim of the study was to teach Mr S to use a notebook to look up information that he could not remember. It was hoped that by using a notebook Mr S would become less reliant on his wife for day-to-day information.

In a number of recent studies, amnesic patients have been trained to use a diary or notebook (Davies & Binks, 1983; Kreutzer, Wehman, Conder & Morrison, 1989; Sohlberg & Mateer, 1989). In each case, diary usage was found to have beneficial effects on daily living. An attempt had been made previously by Mrs S to encourage her husband to use a diary. This attempt had failed, however, because Mr S was resistant to the idea of a diary and had a highly ingrained tendency to rely on his wife for information. In contrast, Mr S could learn new information when motivated to do so. He had, for example, learned how to tune his TV to Sky Channel in order to watch *Star Trek* and he knew what time the programme was on. An important factor in the success of the study was therefore likely to be one of motivation. In order to establish the behaviour of looking up information in a notebook and to try and motivate Mr S, a two-stage approach was adopted. This is consistent with other studies that have used a multi-stage approach to notebook use (e.g. Sohlberg & Mateer, 1989).

In the first stage of the study, Mr S learned a number of novel paired associates and used a notebook to look up responses. The primary aim of this first stage was to establish the habit of looking up information in a notebook. In addition, it was hoped that a demonstration of successful learning using a notebook would help to convince Mr S that the technique was of potential use to him in everyday life. In the second stage of the study, having established the habit of notebook use, we explored whether Mr S could learn to use the notebook in an analogous fashion to access information about real, everyday events. Before and after each stage of the study, Mrs S completed a checklist that detailed her husband's repetitive questioning. This allowed us to establish whether notebook use decreased the extent of Mr S's reliance on his wife for factual information.

CASE HISTORY

Mr S suffered two strokes, the more recent in May 1993. An MRI scan carried out in January 1994 indicated widespread neuropathological changes including a lesion in the posterior limb of the right internal capsule, a lesion in the white matter of the right parietal lobe, and evidence of ischaemic changes compatible with cerebro-vascular disease. Both lateral ventricles and the third ventricle were abnormally large and there was moderate to severe generalised cortical atrophy.

A psychometric assessment was carried out three months after Mr S's stroke and five months before the start of the current study. This revealed a WAIS–R FSIQ of 101 (Verbal 105; Performance 97) which compared reasonably with an estimated premorbid IQ of 111 (Nelson, 1991). On the WMS–R, Mr S had a General Memory Index of 65 and a Delayed Recall Index of 58. This memory deficit covered both verbal and non-verbal material.

Copying of the Rey Figure was 29/36 (10th percentile) and both immediate (1/36) and delayed recall (0/36) were extremely poor. On the five learning trials of the Rey Auditory–Verbal Learning Test (RAVLT), Mr S scored a maximum of 7/15. This fell to 1/15 after the interference trial and 0/15 following a 30-minute delay. On the Warrington Recognition Memory Test (Warrington, 1984) performance was at, or close to, chance on both tasks (Words 28/50; Faces 23/50). On the Wisconsin Card Sorting Test (modified version; Nelson, 1976) Mr S was markedly impaired (2 categories, 21 perseverative errors), and his FAS word fluency (Benton, Hamsher, Varney, & Spreen, 1983) was also significantly reduced (24). Cognitive estimation (Shallice & Evans, 1978) was within normal limits (3). On the Graded Naming Test (McKenna & Warrington, 1983) he scored 22/30 (bright normal range).

A follow-up assessment was carried out 12 months after the initial assessment and one month after completion of the present notebook study. The only notable improvement was an increase in Mr S's WMS–R Visual Memory Index from 64 to 83, with a consequent increase in General Memory Index from 65 to 73. This improvement was largely a reflection of better performance on the Visual Reproduction subtest. But, as Wechsler (1987) points out, the Visual Reproduction subtest has lower reliability relative to other subtests and caution should be applied in interpreting results. Mr S's Attention Index also indicated some improvement (104), but of importance is the fact that his Verbal Index remained the same (75) and his Delay Index showed only minimal improvement (60). Similarly on the RAVLT, the Rey Figure, and the Warrington Recognition Memory Test, Mr S's performance remained very poor. On the WCST and FAS, there was also no sign of improvement. Thus, any decrease in repetitive questioning following the notebook study is unlikely to be accounted for by an improvement in memory or executive functioning.

STAGE 1: ACQUISITION

In Stage 1, Mr S used the notebook to study novel paired associates. These paired associates were studied under two conditions: errorless and errorful learning. It has recently been demonstrated that errorless learning is a more effective method of learning in amnesic patients (Baddeley & Wilson, 1994). Baddeley and Wilson suggest that memory-impaired people rely more on implicit memory when learning new information, but that implicit memory is of little use in correcting errors once erroneous responses have been made. Thus, a teaching method that prevents the introduction of errors should be more effective than a method where errors are plentiful. A notebook seemed an ideal medium in which to compare errorless and errorful learning.

In addition to establishing the behaviour of notebook use, it was hoped that Mr S would gradually learn the information in his notebook. This demonstration of learning could then be used as an additional form of motivation to encourage Mr S to take part in Stage 2, the application of the notebook to daily events.

Method

Before initiation of the notebook training, Mrs S completed a daily checklist for 23 days. Each day she recorded all instances on which Mr S asked her for information. She noted down each question and put a tick against one each time it was asked. The 23-day period constituted a training period during which it was ensured that Mrs S understood the task and was complying with the instructions. Following the training period, Mrs S filled in the checklist consistently for seven days. This gave a baseline measure of Mr S's repetitive questioning and provided information about the type of questions that might be addressed by Stage 2 of the study.

Materials. Forty pictures taken from the Snodgrass and Vanderwart (1980) norms were paired in a pseudo-random fashion: no pair members began with the same letter or were from the same semantic category. The materials were piloted on a group of eight control subjects in order to establish the ease with which each association could be learned. Each subject was presented with the 20 picture pairs in random order at a rate of one every three seconds. Each picture pair was presented on a 5" × 3" index card. After presentation of all 20 pairs, subjects were presented with test cards. A test card contained the first picture of a pair, and subjects were asked to name the picture that had been paired with the one shown. Errors were corrected verbally. After testing on all 20 pairs, subjects were tested a second and a third time (with no further presentation of the original picture pairs). On each trial, the test cards were presented one at a time in random order. Subjects were given verbal feedback and corrected where necessary. Finally, subjects were tested once more following a delay of two hours. Using data from both immediate and delayed testing, two lists of equal difficulty were created. Each list comprised 10 picture pairs. One list was designated for errorless learning and the other for errorful learning.

The 20 pairs of target pictures were placed in a small notebook, one pair to a page. Test cards had the first picture only on them, and were coded on the back for the errorful or errorless condition. Each page of the notebook was numbered sequentially. This page number corresponded to the number on the back of the test card for that pair.

Procedure. In the first session of the notebook training, Mr S was told that he would be learning to make associations between pairs of pictures. He was shown one member of a pair and was required to say which picture was paired in his notebook with the one shown. For some of the pairs he was asked to make a guess at the answer, and for others he was asked to look up the answer immediately in his notebook. The instructions for the errorful and errorless conditions were as follows:

Errorful instructions: "I want you to look at this picture and try to remember (or *guess* for first presentation) which picture goes with it, you can have three tries." After three tries: "You can look up the answer now—it is picture number X in your book. Look at the two pictures together, and try to remember them for next time."

Errorless instructions: "I want you to look up the picture that goes with this one, don't guess. It is picture number *X* in your book. Look at the two pictures together, and try to remember them for next time."

The test cards were presented in random order. Thus, errorful and errorless items were randomly interspersed. The procedure was repeated twice so that Mr S saw each picture pair three times in a session. A different random order of presentation was used on each trial. Notebook training was continued for 10 sessions over a period of 16 days. During these training sessions only the errorless and errorful procedures indicated earlier were carried out: there was no additional free or cued recall during this period. In Session 10, there were only two training presentations of each pair. Following the second presentation, an immediate cued recall test for all pairs was carried out. The 20 test cards were presented with the following instruction: "I am going to show you a picture and I would like you to tell me which picture went with it in your notebook."

Using the same cued recall test procedure, Mr S had three further test sessions at delays of 24 hours, 7 days, and 10 weeks. In the 24-hour delay session, Mr S was given three consecutive test trials. Five minutes later he was given another three consecutive test trials. After a further 15 minutes he was given one more test trial. In both the 7-day and 10-week delay sessions, Mr S was given three consecutive test trials. These tests enabled measurements to be made of both between-sessions and within-session recall after various delays. In all test trials, Mr S was shown a picture and was required to recall which picture went with that one in his notebook. He was informed whether his answer was correct and, if it was not, the correct answer was provided verbally.

At the end of Stage 1 of the study, the checklist procedure was repeated for seven days to determine whether there had been any change in Mr S's repetitive questioning. The purpose of this intermediate checklist was to ascertain whether any reduction in repetitive questioning at the end of the study could be attributed to Mr S merely having regular visits from the experimenter. (Data were only available for six of the seven days in this designated checklist period.)

Results

The results of the acquisition stage of the study are shown in Table 11.1. The data show a very clear superiority for the errorless learning method in that, consistently, more items are recalled in the errorless condition than in the errorful condition. A Sign Test indicated that the superiority of errorless over errorful learning was significant ($P < .0005$). On immediate test, a measurement of within-session retention, twice as many correct responses were produced following errorless learning. The repetition of cued recall tests across and within sessions allowed further measurement of both between-sessions and within-session retention following various delays. For neither method was there a high level of between-sessions retention. After 24 hours only one item in each condition was recalled initially although, after a seven-day delay, 50% of learned items in the errorless condition were recalled. For both methods there was an improvement in retention within a session. The size of this improvement (e.g. 5/6 correct on the second trial in the 24-hour delay) suggested that Mr S showed savings from previous sessions that had not been initially apparent. Furthermore, not only were more items recalled following errorless learning, but on average a greater proportion of learned items were produced following errorless learning (62%) than following errorful learning (55%)

The results from the checklist are shown in Table 11.2. To simplify the analysis, questions on the checklist were divided into four categories: recent events, events today, future events, and other. The overall extent of Mr S's questioning before and after Stage 1 of the study showed a small increase: a fall in number of questions about future events was offset by an increase in number of questions about recent events and events today.

Discussion of Stage 1

It was demonstrated in Stage 1 that Mr S could learn novel associations and that this learning was more effective when an errorless learning procedure was used. These data are consistent with other studies that have shown a superiority for errorless learning. Wilson, Baddeley, Evans, and Shiel (1994) found that errorless learning promoted retention on a range of tasks including remembering word lists, relearning the names of objects, and learning the names of hospital staff. It is particularly important that Wilson et al.'s study, along with the current study, demonstrates that errorless learning can facilitate the acquisition of novel associations, because it is this aspect of learning that is particularly difficult for memory-disordered patients.

TABLE 11.1
Number of Paired Associates Correctly Recalled
by Mr S as a Function of Errorless
vs Errorful Learning

	Errorless	Errorful	Total
Immediate	6	3	9
24 hour delay	1	1	2
	5	3	8
	4	2	6
(5 min delay)	4	1	5
	6	2	8
	4	4	8
(15 min delay)	4	1	5
7 day delay	3	0	3
	4	2	6
	6	1	7
10 week delay	1	1	2
	2	1	3
	2	1	3

TABLE 11.2
Checklist Scores Indicating Mean Number of Questions per
Day Asked by Mr S at Different Stages of the Study

	Baseline	After Stage 1	After Stage 2
Recent	0	1.33 (1.63) (Range 0–4)	0
Today	4.71 (1.80) (Range 3–8)	6.00 (4.00) (Range 1–12)	2.71 (2.36) (Range 1–6)
Future	2.71 (2.43) (Range 2–7)	0	1.43 (1.81) (Range 0–4)
Other	0.57 (1.51) (Range 0–4)	0.83 (1.33) (Range 0–3)	1.71 (2.43) (Range 0–6)
Total	7.99	8.16	5.85

Standard deviations in parentheses.

In terms of repetitive questioning, Mr S appeared to show a decrease in number of questions about future events but an increase in those about recent events and events today. It is inevitable that these types of data are noisy, but it should be noted that, for the area specified by Mrs S as being particularly problematic (events today), there was no reduction.

STAGE 2: APPLICATION

In Stage 1 we achieved the primary aim of familiarising Mr S with the use of a notebook as a means of accessing information. Indeed it was noticeable that in the first study he quickly began asking if he could look up the answer when he did not know it. We had thus demonstrated to Mr S the ease with which he could look up information in his notebook. Furthermore, he was able to remember some of this information, particularly that learned under errorless conditions. We were therefore able to convince Mr S that a notebook had potential for everyday use.

Stage 2 was aimed at generalising the use of a notebook to Mr S's personal situation. Completion of the checklists by Mrs S provided a baseline indication of Mr S's repetitive questioning from which the value of any intervention could be judged. The errorless learning paradigm used in Stage 1 was adapted to allow us to train Mr S to look up facts about daily events.

Method

Procedure.   Diary entries of the day's, or week's, events were made in a small notebook (e.g. visits, visitors, meals, items of interest etc.). These entries were intended to cover the areas identified by the checklist filled out by Mrs S, but those most frequently entered were those relating to recent events and events today (e.g. 2.00pm today: Chiropodist). Mr S was encouraged to make these entries daily with the help of Mrs S for prompts. In each session, 10 diary entries were selected. The entries were allocated a number (1–10) and Mr S was asked questions relating to each one (e.g. Where are you going at two o'clock this afternoon?). Mr S was required to look up the answer to the question each time. This ensured that the method mimicked the errorless condition in Stage 1. Each diary entry was addressed three times in a session, and the order of questioning was random. The schedule for Stage 2 was as follows:

Week 1 – 3 visits
Week 2 – 2 visits
Week 3 – 2 visits
Week 4 – 1 visit

At the end of Stage 2, the checklist was completed again for seven days to assess whether the study had made a significant difference to Mr S's dependence on Mrs S for information that he could obtain for himself.

Results

Table 11.2 shows the checklist scores obtained after the notebook training programme. The success of notebook training was measured by comparing the results of the post-Stage 2 checklist with those of the checklist completed at the outset of the study. In terms of total questioning there was a reduction relative to the initial baseline. The number of questions about recent events returned to the baseline level of zero, questions about events today were reduced by 42%, and those about future events were reduced by 47%. This was offset by an increase in questions categorised as "other". The statistical significance of the overall reduction in questioning was assessed using related t-tests, with days as the random factor. (Autocorrelational analyses indicated that Mr S's questioning on successive days did not show significant serial dependency, e.g. Kazdin, 1982. It is assumed, therefore, that the data are uncorrelated over time and that the use of t-tests is appropriate.) The reduction in overall questioning was significant, $t(6)=2.29$, $P < .04$. More detailed analysis revealed that most of the reduction in questioning could be accounted for by a reduction in *repetitiveness* as opposed to Mr S asking a smaller range of questions. This breakdown of the data is shown in Table 11.3. There was no difference between the number of different questions asked before and after notebook training ($P > .4$), but there was a significant reduction in repetitiveness, i.e. number of times that Mr S asked a question that he had already asked on a particular day, $t(6)=4.04$, $P < .004$. This represented a decrease of 57% and 54% in "today" and "future" questions, respectively, relative to the initial baseline.

TABLE 11.3
Checklist Scores Showing Mean Number of Different Questions and Mean Number of Repeated Questions per Day

	Baseline	After Stage 1	After Stage 2
New questions	2.43 (0.79)	3.17 (1.47)	2.57 (1.27)
Repeated questions	5.57 (1.62)	5.00 (2.90)	3.29 (1.60)

Standard deviations in parentheses.

Discussion of Stage 2

Notebook training was effective in reducing the number of times that Mr S asked questions about daily events. On subsequent unannounced visits, Mr S was still using his notebook, although he does depend on Mrs S making the diary entries each day. Mrs S reported that if she had not completed the entries first thing in the morning, Mr S states that he will not know "where he is". Both Mr and Mrs S felt that the study had been a success, and that Mr S would continue to use the notebook and find it useful.

GENERAL DISCUSSION

Stage 1 of the study demonstrated that an errorless learning procedure can be used to teach novel associations. Stage 2 showed that the use of a notebook, behaviour acquired in Stage 1, was applicable to daily events. Moreover, notebook use led to a reduction in repetitive questions about these events.

It is acknowledged that this single-case design is essentially an exploratory study. However, attention is drawn to the follow-up psychometric data, which indicate that a reduction in repetitive questioning cannot be accounted for by any improvement in memory or executive functioning. Furthermore, it is important to note that there was only a reduction in questioning rate about daily events, i.e. events targeted in the notebook. Other types of questioning (e.g. how are you? did you sleep well?) continued to be about the same. This indicated that the training had a rather specific effect. For repetitive questioning to be reduced further it is suggested that the notebook method is extended to include other classes of information. This remains a plausible option for future intervention.

In sum, this study showed how an initially difficult and highly dependent patient can be "educated by stealth" into the use of a notebook, which then has a positive influence on his actual daily behaviour. It is hoped that future studies of rehabilitation might develop this approach along with other recent strategies adopted for notebook and diary training (e.g. Sohlberg & Mateer, 1989).

More recent follow-up visits have revealed that Mr S is no longer using the notebook. Mrs S reported that she had taken over the task of filling in the notebook as she found this to be simpler than providing Mr S with the information. At the outset it was thought to be desirable for Mr S to complete the diary entries himself, as this would serve to reinforce his sense of self-reliance and establish a behaviour that would enable him to continue without the assistance of Mrs S. Unfortunately, Mrs S has now discontinued filling in the diary entries. This highlights the importance of motivation and commitment from all parties when embarking on any rehabilitation strategy, and suggests that fostering the appropriate locus of control is essential.

The first stage of the notebook study provided a basis for further research into errorless learning and the use of explicit and implicit memory in memory-impaired individuals. To assess the generality of the errorless learning advantage in the acquisition of novel associations, we have recently carried out two group studies of verbal association learning (Squires, Hunkin, & Parkin, 1997). Each study involved 16 memory-impaired subjects and, in both studies, half the associations were taught by an errorless method and half were taught by an errorful method. In the first study, we compared the effectiveness of the two methods when subjects were required to learn associations that were remotely linked (e.g. menu – pepper) and in the second study we compared the effectiveness of the two methods in the acquisition of totally novel associations. In both studies, subjects showed an advantage for items learned by the errorless method and this was most pronounced for learning novel associations. On these grounds it would seem that errorless learning is an effective means of helping memory-impaired patients acquire novel associations and we are hopeful that this method can be effectively transferred to the rehabilitation setting.

In contrast to our findings, Evans et al. (submitted) have found more limited success in the use of errorless learning. They recently investigated the effectiveness of errorless and errorful learning in identifying degraded pictures, learning names, learning a route, and programming an electronic aid. They describe three studies involving 10 separate experiments comparing two errorless methods with a trial-and-error method. They found an advantage for errorless learning in face–name learning when subjects were cued with a photograph of the face and the initial letter of the name. However, they found no advantage for errorless learning in face–name free recall, when subjects were only given the photograph of the face to name. On other tasks they did not demonstrate an advantage for errorless learning, and on one task they found an advantage for trial-and-error learning (route learning). Correlational analysis carried out by the authors suggested that those subjects who benefited more from the errorless procedure were more severely memory impaired when tested on the Rivermead Behavioural Memory Test. They suggest that the more the individual has to rely on implicit memory, the greater the gain derived from the errorless technique, and conclude that errorless learning is mediated by reducing interference with implicit memory, thereby enabling those with greater memory impairments to benefit more from errorless learning. They propose that errorless learning may only be effective for tasks in which implicit memory can be used to strengthen pre-existing associations (e.g. learning names in response to a first letter cue), and is generally ineffective for tasks that require novel association learning (e.g. route learning, using an electronic organiser, and learning names where the first letter cue was not available).

Our notebook study and our later (Squires et al., 1997) study, contradict this conclusion, as a greater advantage was observed for novel associations than for words for which there was a pre-existing connection. One possible explanation for the contradictions between our findings and those of Evans et al. (submitted) could be differences in the amount of effort/active participation involved during learning. Jones and Eyres (1992) highlight the problem of passivity during learning in which errors are avoided, but this problem was taken into consideration both by ourselves and by Evans et al., in that attempts were made to incorporate active participation in every task. As the tasks used in the different studies were not equivalent, it is nonetheless possible that different levels of active participation occurred. For example, the Squires et al. procedure required subjects to find an association for the verbally presented cue and response words, and to write the two words down. The act of converting phonologically coded information into orthographic form may provide sufficient additional processing for information to be more easily retained (Conway & Gathercole, 1990). However, as verbally presented words were also written down in the errorful method it is not clear why this should convey an additional advantage for errorless learning. Evans et al. also incorporated writing in their procedure for face–name learning, which, interestingly, did show a significant advantage for errorless learning in two of the three experiments carried out. The one experiment where the advantage was not present (Study 2) required subjects to carry out a free recall test before cued recall, which meant that errors were introduced before the cued recall trials in both conditions. Writing was not part of the procedure for our notebook study, but this was carried out over repeated sessions and the additional exposure to the stimuli probably outweighed any advantage conferred by writing during only one session.

Another possible explanation for the different results observed could be one of application. Evans et al. have applied the methods to naturalistic procedures that are more complicated than the experimental procedure used by ourselves. It is possible that errorless learning confers an advantage in an experimental setting but is not well suited to more realistic tasks. This is an important issue, as the aim of the research is to find a method of learning that will facilitate learning in memory-impaired individuals to enable them to lead more fulfilling lives. We would suggest that although the method does appear to have potential for use in a rehabilitation setting, it needs more detailed investigation before it can be successfully applied to more complicated tasks of the type required in everyday life.

ACKNOWLEDGEMENTS

This work was partly funded by the Wellcome Trust (Grant number 037666/Z/93/Z/ 1.4U) and the MRC. We thank Mr and Mrs S. for their co-operation in this study.

REFERENCES

Baddeley, A., & Wilson, B.A. (1994). When implicit learning fails: Amnesia and the problem of error elimination. *Neuropsychologia, 92*, 53–68.

Benton, A.L., Hamsher, K., Varney, N., & Spreen, O. (1983). *Contributions to neuropsychological assessment.* New York: Oxford University Press.

Conway, M.A., & Gathercole, S.E. (1990). Writing and long-term memory: Evidence for a "Translation" hypothesis. *The Quarterly Journal of Experimental Psychology, 42A*, 513–527.

Davies, A.D.M., & Binks, M.G. (1983). Supporting the residual memory of a Korsakoff patient. *Behavioural Psychotherapy, 11*, 62–74.

Evans, J.J., Wilson, B.A., Schuri, U., Baddeley, A., Canavan, T., Laaksonen, R., Bruna, O., Lorenzi, L., Della Sala, S., Andrade, J., Green, R., & Taussik, I. (submitted). A comparison of 'errorless' and 'trial and error' learning methods for teaching individuals with acquired memory deficits. *Neuropsychological Rehabilitation.*

Jones, R.S.P., & Eyres, C.B. (1992). The use of errorless learning procedures in teaching people with a learning disability: A critical review. *Mental Handicap Research, 5*, 204–212.

Kazdin, A.E. (1982). *Single-case research designs: Methods for clinical and applied settings.* Oxford University Press.

Kreutzer, J., Wehman, P., Conder, R., & Morrison, C. (1989). Compensatory strategies for enhancing living and vocational outcome following traumatic brain injury. *Cognitive Rehabilitation, 9*, 30–35.

McKenna, P., & Warrington, E.K. (1983). *Graded Naming Test.* London: NFER–Nelson.

Nelson, H.E. (1976). A modified card sorting test sensitive to frontal lobe defects. *Cortex, 12*, 313–324.

Nelson, H.E. (1991). *National Adult Reading Test* (2nd Edn.) London: NFER–Nelson.

Shallice, T. & Evans, M. (1978). The involvement of the frontal lobes in cognitive estimation. *Cortex, 14*, 294–303.

Snodgrass, J.G., & Vanderwart, M. (1980). A standardised set of 260 pictures: Norms for name agreement, image agreement, familiarity and visual complexity. *Journal of Experimental Psychology: Human Learning and Memory, 6*, 174–215.

Sohlberg, M.M., & Mateer, C.A. (1989). Training use of compensatory memory books: A three stage behavioural approach. *Journal of Clinical and Experimental Neuropsychology, 11*, 871–879.

Squires, E.J., Hunkin, N.M., & Parkin, A.J. (1997). Can errorless learning facilitate the learning of novel associations in amnesia? *Neuropsychologia.*

Warrington, E.K. (1984). *Recognition Memory Test.* London: NFER–Nelson.

Wechsler, D. (1987). *The Wechsler Memory Scale–Revised.* San Antonio, CA: The Psychological Corporation.

Wilson, B.A., Baddeley, A.D., Evans, J., & Shiel, A. (1994). Errorless learning in the rehabilitation of memory impaired people. *Neuropsychological Rehabilitation, 4*, 307–326.

Wilson, B.A., Cockburn, J., & Baddeley, A. (1985). *The Rivermead Behavioural Memory Test.* Reading, UK: Thames Valley Test Company.

Author Index

Goldman-Rakic, P.S., 158
Goldstein, G., 142
Goodglass, H., 71, 94
Gottesman, I.I., 142, 154
Grady, C.L., 11
Graham, D.I., 58
Graham, K.S., 84–5, 88, 98–9, 101
Grasby, P.M., 70
Grattan, L.M., 131
Greenwood, R.J., 189
Grossi, D., 71
Guildford, J.P., 131
Gur, R.C., 155
Gur, R.E., 155

Haist, F., 57
Hall, K.M., 189
Hamsher, K., 65, 90, 131, 148, 193
Hanley, J.R., 71, 112, 117, 121–3, 137
Harlow, J.M., 127–8
Harsent, L., 132
Harvey, I., 154
Heaton, R.K., 142
Heggs, A.J., 107
Hellawell, D.J., 166
Hillis, A.E., 100, 106
Hirsch, S.R., 142, 155
Hodges, J., 18, 20, 26, 37, 75, 84–7, 92, 96–7, 99, 101, 106–7
Hollingworth, H.L., 115
Hollows, S., 42, 46
Holzman, P.S., 158
Howard, D., 86, 100, 153
Humber, S.A., 152
Humphreys, G.W., 106, 153
Hunkin, N.M., 64–9, 73, 159, 175, 201
Huppert, F.A., 175

Issac, C., 22

Jacoby, L.L., 115
Java, R.I., 133
Johnson, K.L., 142
Johnstone, E.C., 142
Jones, R.S.P., 202
Joseph, A.B., 175

Jus, A., 59
Jus, K., 59

Kamphurst, W., 84
Kaney, S., 166
Kaplan, E., 71, 94
Kapur, N., 3, 37, 57, 59, 63, 75, 77–9
Kapur, S., 14
Karbe, H., 84
Kavanagh, D.J., 156
Kay, J., 89, 97
Kazdin, A.E., 199
Kennedy, P., 59, 75
Kertesz, A., 84
Kervetz, A., 148
Kime, S.K., 180
King, D.J., 156
Kolb, B., 157
Kopelman, M.D., 46, 48, 50, 56, 66, 169, 175
Kotapka, M.J., 58
Kraeplin, E., 142, 160
Kreutzer, J., 192
Kritchevsky, M., 57
Kuipers, L., 155

Lamb, D.G., 160
Landauer, T.K., 182
Laws, K.R., 152, 160
Leafhead, K.M., 165–7, 175–6
Leber, W.R., 131
Leff, J.P., 142, 155
Lencz, T., 9
Leng, N.R.C., 3, 66, 121, 128, 175
Leonard, G., 124
Lerer, B., 157
Lesser, R., 89
Levasseur, M., 10
Lewis, S.W., 155
Liddle, P.F., 142, 155, 157
Light, R.H., 131
Liotti, M., 57
Longmore, B.E., 65
Luchelli, M., 38, 64, 74, 79
Luzzatti, C., 84

Subject Index

abstract designs test, 132–3
affordances, 106
Alphabet Test, 70
anomia, 86–9
anterior communicating artery aneurysm, 3, 112, 128
anterior thalamus, 18
anterograde amnesia, 21–4, 28–9, 99–100, 111–115
autobiographical amnesia, 40–42, 45–50, 52, 54–6, 57–60, 78
see also retrograde amnesia
autobiographical memory interview (AMI), 46, 56, 68
   vs. public knowledge, 78

binding code, 76
BOLD, 9

Calev matched recall and recognition test, 24–5, 28, 114–5
Capgras Syndrome, 4
Celebrity Faces Test, 71
Clocks Test, 71
Cognitive Esimates Test, 29, 32, 131, 150
colloid cyst, 15
computerised tomography (CT), 7–8
confabulation, 112, 129–130
convergence zones, 76
Cookie Theft Picture, 94
Cotard's delusion, 4, 129–130
   facial memory, 171–3

memory for buildings, 173–4
theories, 165–7, 174–6

description vs. verification, 121–2, 137
Doors and People Test, 21–22

Ekman & Friesen faces, 173
encoding deficits, 113–4, 137–9
errorful learning, 193
errorless learning, 193–200
external memory aids, 179–82
   see also JC's system

FAIR, 9
false alarms, 24, 132, 135–9
feature code, 77
focal retrograde amnesia, 2, 63–4
focused retrieval deficit, 122–3, 136
fornix, 18–20, 25
frontal lobes
   memory disorders, 32–3, 111–124, 127–139
functional magnetic resonance imaging (fMRI), 8–11

Gage, Phineas, 127–8

head injury, 48–59, 64–5
Herpes Simplex encephalitis, 7–8
hippocampus, 8, 18

imagery, 70–72
index codes, 77
intrusion errors, 130–131

For Product Safety Concerns and Information please contact our EU
representative GPSR@taylorandfrancis.com Taylor & Francis Verlag GmbH,
Kaufingerstraße 24, 80331 München, Germany

Printed and bound by CPI Group (UK) Ltd, Croydon, CR0 4YY

08/06/2025
01896985-0006